BREAST CANCER!

You're kidding...right?

BREAST CANCER!

You're kidding...right?

LIVING LIFE THROUGH THE PRISM OF UNCERTAINTY AND HAVING A GOOD TIME!

CATHERINE DOUGHTY, MS, CCHI

THREE ARROW PUBLISHING

Published by Three Arrow Publishing
ISBN: 978-0-615-49859-1
Library of Congress Control Number: 2011941977

Book design by Brion Sausser

TABLE OF CONTENTS

ACKNOWLEDGEMENTS

I have the privilege of being the mother of two exceptional children. Stephanie and Tommie, you are the loves of my life and my constant source of inspiration. I love you to the core of my being, and want you both to know that when all this cancer was happening, you guys were young, innocent and unaware. The two of you were the reason I sought healing and understanding, so that I could live with you, and most importantly continue to be your mother, your mentor, and on occasion when you needed it, your manhandler! You two keep me together, whole and strong, and the love I have for you, is what pulled me through. Know this; from the day you both were born, and opened your eyes for the first time, it has been nothing short of a miracle to watch you unfold.

I dedicate this book to you both, to my family, and friends. Your love and devotion through my experience in navigating cancer, and living life through the prism of uncertainty enabled me to write this book.

Special thanks to Cynthia Huijgens, M.Ed., who served as my copy editor and proofreader and helped me make sense of wording and phrases. Kelli R. Trungale, MLS, ELS, who served as my medical editor. You both were instrumental in shepherding the project to completion.

Also, a hug to Brion Sausser at www.BookCreatives.com who worked his infinite supply of brilliance and creative genius capturing the essence of what I desired for the cover and interior design of the book; it is alive, sexy, serious and a lot of fun. The esteemed gratitude I have for your commitment to the project goes beyond words.

PREFACE

The content presented in this book derives from my actual experience as a breast cancer patient and survivor. At the time of my diagnosis in 2007, I was separated from my husband after two decades of marriage. I had two small children ages six and nine. I was working full time as a hospital department director, was nearly halfway through a graduate degree program in biomedical informatics, and enjoying weekly workouts at my local YMCA. One of my passions was playing guitar in a band on Sundays during praise and worship services at my Lutheran church.

At the time of the cancer diagnosis, my life was satisfying and rich. Looking back, I felt at the top of my game. I have always been fiercely independent and consider myself competent in everything I do, but when I discovered I had cancer, I didn't have the slightest idea of what to do. I needed to navigate the medical maze quickly as a cancer patient who quite honestly, more than wanting to be cured and healed from cancer forever, just wanted to look sexually attractive, naked to the heterosexual male. Once the reality of having breast cancer sunk in, and I had moved beyond being scared and shocked, I could not deny that the best outcome for me was to stay alive and have fabulous-looking breasts.

OK, wait a minute! Let me explain my motivation in greater detail so you don't think that my vanity overruled my desire to be present for my children, and continue living my full and satisfying life. The truth of the matter was, focusing on what I truly wanted in the end, and not just surfacing from the experience as a "survivor," was deeply empowering. I absolutely didn't know what to do or how to do it when I was informed about the disease, but I definitively knew that cancer was not going to rob me of my, femininity or life, and for me, that included large, voluptuous breasts.

Each disappointing medical encounter I experienced during my journey, further fueled my determination to seek the best medical expertise available, while strategizing my surgical and treatment options. I spent a lot of time developing a well thought out plan of care I would ultimately implement, in order to direct and control my recovery. By not allowing myself to succumb to the disease, and wanting to emerge from cancer with two beautiful breasts and a cancer-free smoking-hot body—I had the motivation to search out and partner with the expertise that would yield the results I wanted.

This book chronicles my experience and tries to convey the lessons cancer taught me. You will find that my cancer case was perhaps a little more complicated than most in that I had endured a breast surgery weeks prior. Indeed, it was during this first surgery that the cancer was found. At the time, I had a lot of questions, and found myself spiraling in a thousand different directions, down a thousand different holes; until it occurred to me that what I needed in order to make sense of this unbelievable situation already existed inside me. Through my professional experiences as a Director of Diagnostic and Interventional Imaging with Lean Six Sigma Black Belt training, I knew there was a proven methodology that could help me make focused clinical decisions in an uncertain decision space. With this new clarity of mind, I refocused my energies; and created tools that gave me a strategic approach to navigating the medical maze. I prayed for wisdom continually, and utilized what I already knew. And you know what? It helped tremendously.

In this book, I am going to share with you not only how I approached each medical decision with calm and confidence, keeping my eye on the goal, but also how my experience with cancer put my life back on a directional course quickly—a new and improved one that would begin my understanding of the prism of uncertainty.

As a prologue to my story, I have created forms and discussion documents for you to utilize during your medical consultations. These will enable you to have a very organized approach as you meet with your specialty and subspecialty experts, with whom you will ultimately consent to surgery and treatment with. I have attempted to take very theoretical clinical processes, and simplified them in a methodology you can apply in very practical terms to the phases of a cancer diagnosis and treatment as you experience them.

My name is Catherine L. Doughty, MS, CCHI. I read informatics journal articles, do frequency analyses, finance, make charts and statistical tables. I have LED lights in my cateyed reading glasses, but don't be fooled. I am a tall, sexy, and intelligent individual who prides herself on the ability to create viable solutions for individuals and institutions, and likes to be called Cathy or Cat. I have created my own character in this book, and I named her the Cancer Cat. She will be your go-to girl for life-saving, critical thinking and strategic advice to enable you to easily navigate your way through the medical maze and get your life back in control.

Throughout each chapter, I have included Cancer Cat Advice and Cancer Cat Tips as well as recaps for each phase of scientific methodology. Use this information to the max! These are valuable tools for those who are struggling as I did, to focus on a forward moving approach that is likely to yield the best results. You will need to read, review and consider each point as it applies to you and your treatment process. This Cancer Cat wants you to enjoy and live all nine of your lives, but most especially this one, and evolve into the magnificent creature you were born to be. So stay with me, because you're about to receive the conduit to the catnip for your cancer diagnosis and learn how to seek the clinical expertise required for a spectacular and satisfying outcome with breast cancer. You can visit my website at www.The Cancer Cat.com.

I am honored you have chosen to read my book, and my

very best wishes are with you as you continue your journey from a cancer diagnosis to the other side of life. My hope is that you will feel empowered and be able to move quickly through the initial shock from the cancer challenges, recognize your own wisdom and intelligence, and look absolutely beautiful. It's the living end, I promise you!

SEEING LIFE THROUGH A PRISM

A prism is a medium that misrepresents or distorts whatever is seen thorough it. According to Merriam-Webster, uncertainty is a situation in which the current state of knowledge is such that (1) the order or nature of things is unknown; (2) the consequences, extent, or magnitude of circumstances, conditions, or events is unpredictable; and (3) credible probabilities to possible outcomes cannot be assigned. Although too much uncertainty is undesirable, manageable uncertainty provides the freedom to make creative decisions. You may be asking, "How do you acquire the skill set to make uncertainty manageable?" This question is difficult to answer in business situations, let alone in personal life-threatening ones where your life is at risk.

I had a life-threatening illness with a lot of uncertainties, and what I thought I was looking at continued to be misrepresented. What I determined later was that the cancer had been there in my big, beautiful breast for years prior to its discovery—it didn't just appear overnight, so the day before I was diagnosed was no different than the day prior, I just had no knowledge of cancer in my body. I was blissfully unaware! The day I came to know with certainty I had cancer was the day I felt I had to start navigating my way through it, again another misrepresentation because it had been there for years. Cancer became my prism!

As I lost my breasts (nipples and all!), my reproductivity, my hair, my six-figure job, my physical strength, and my marriage, I sunk deeper into uncertainty. Each time I lost something I hoped I had hit the bottom of that big black hole I was spiraling down. Every time I lost a bit more of myself, I would ask the question, "How much further can I descend? When I refocused my thoughts, I would answer the question with, "You're going to go as far as it takes!" I made myself wake up and see life as it really is, to understand that this experience today is only one group of moments in the here and now of a very happy, successful, and fulfilling life. I forced myself to love every sexy second of my life—even disappointing news, and unsatisfactory recommendations from professionals I admired and respected. I vowed to keep my sense of humor intact, and have a good time in the interim, no matter how I felt. This is how I came to face my fear of uncertainty.

One thing my training as a Director of Diagnostic and Interventional Imaging and a Lean Six Sigma Black Belt, in the healthcare industry taught me is that imaging, pathology and data are integral and pivotal components in organizing the decision-making process when it comes to a cancer diagnosis. It also has statistical significance on the plan of care that both a clinician recommends and a patient ultimately decides upon executing. I also learned that no matter how philosophical you are, you cannot control any reaction when the rug keeps getting pulled out from underneath you. The truth is, the rug isn't being pulled out from under you; it just seems that way, which is another misrepresentation. A more helpful and focused un-derstanding is to see each piece of information as exactly what you need to spiral up, and work out your plan of care. Take this opportunity to call upon the knowledge already inside you, and experience the growth required for your cancer journey and the next phase of your life.

During the beginning of my diagnosis, I responded with fear many times and would circle back to meet with others on and off the path who helped me see the possibilities of change, and the value of scientific methodology in my own way of think-ing and coping. Often, I found myself struggling with my black-and-white perspectives and couldn't control my emotions and my reactions to uncertainty. For a mathematician, twelve times twelve always equals one hundred and forty four, never one hun-dred and forty three. The certainty of the law of addition con-firms that. Time and time again, I took my knowledge and used simple tables and charts to keep me on task as I was interviewing multiple specialists trying to remedy my "little situation." At the time, I was first diagnosed; I found it all so distressing I couldn't even say the word "cancer." However, as I remained focused on my objectives to solve my cancer problem, and began to navigate the medical maze, I felt calm and unshaken when utilizing my materials and staying on the merits, resisting the negative ten-dency to deviate from the goal and becoming sidetracked. Using the methodology allowed me to say the word "cancer" without trepidation, or paralyzing fear. Once I got my head in the right place I emerged triumphant, strong and stunning.

For those of you who have been diagnosed with breast cancer or know of someone who has been diagnosed, my advice to you is, learn everything you can about what is available to you. I have been through most all of it. I had six surgeries within fifteen months, chemotherapy, and radiation. I had immediate free-flap reconstruction at the time of my bilateral mastectomies. Throughout my treatment, I continued to work; I finished a master's degree, got divorced and fired from my job. Within a few weeks following that, I bought a house, continued to parent my children, was gainfully employed again, and recovered my life in the process. So, yes, I have felt the horror, anger, shame, the humiliation, the hurt, and the most unspeakable pain and grief that you may be experiencing right now. I've experienced pride, lust, humor, courage, acceptance and peace from being dealt the cancer card as well. Throughout, I felt determined and hopeful. I believe you can too!

THREE LITTLE WORDS

The three dreaded words no one wants to hear: "You have cancer!" Nobody ever believes the diagnosis is right, not upon hearing it for the first time. It's always somebody else, not me! I certainly didn't believe it, and I kept yelling at the people talking that night about the findings. I thought I was either high, or there had to have been a mistake, or the surgeons were just wrong. This couldn't be happening, but it turned out it was. All I could think at the time was, I had to get it together quickly, and I mean fast. I had two little kids and a mortgage, my marriage was in the trashcan, and now I had a serious life-threatening situation to deal with. What was I going to do?

When I learned of my diagnosis, I was working as a Lean Six Sigma Black Belt for a large Houston hospital. In my position, I reviewed processes and evaluated data to organize a change management plan to improve efficiencies in workflows, and patient outcomes, along with other responsibilities. After the shock of my diagnosis, and considerable searching, I decided the best tools I had in my tool box were the scientific ones I used in my work. As you will discover for yourself, by defining the problem, measuring it, analyzing it, and implementing an improvement solution, you can get your life in and under control more timely.

I will show you an easy step-by-step process which covers all the critical x's or issues impeding your current health status. These are practical, principled items that you need to address with your physicians. These tools will enable you to determine your goals, develop a plan that you can implement and achieve. With Cancer Cat's support you will have the tools required to select a world class medical team, leverage knowledge about your type of cancer, identify potential problems and solve them along the way.

I'm not going to lie to you. When I was going through it, was it easy? No! I was horrified, scared out of my wits, confused and trying to get in touch with specialists, so I could get to the expertise and information I needed to begin to sort it all out. It would have been easier if I had this book and Cancer Cat's information at my fingertips from the beginning to help solve my "little situation," but I didn't. I had to go to multiple sources to do my research, and set up my meetings, create forms and discussion documents to stay on topic and track. It was hard for me, despite being in the health care industry for all of my professional life. If I hadn't had the background I had, who knows where I would be today. And that's why I've written this book. I recognize I had an advantage, and by sharing my account and findings, I hope to level the playing field for you.

First things first, you will need to begin to put together your medical team—a world-class one at that, better than the best of the best! With the exception of my own background and knowledge (which I am passing onto you), I had little support, but the support I had was outstanding. I can't stress enough how important it will be for you to form your own alliances with subject matter experts, world-class clinicians, and individuals who will assist you because you will need them. No matter where you are in the world, there are pockets of expertise to tap into. If you are having difficulty locating professionals in your area, get on the internet and determine the best cancer treatment center proximal to you. Ask for recommendations from individuals who have been where you are now, most will gladly share their learnings if you have time to listen.

For right now, this second, quit worrying! I know you're overwhelmed, exhausted, and sick and tired of crying all night from this nerve-shattering news. I also know you want to run away. You're scared to death that you're going to leave your children motherless or fatherless and your business unfinished, not to mention the possibility of your prosperity on the table for someone else to spend (like your soon-to-be ex-spouse, possibly?). Don't believe it for a second! Not you, baby! Cancer is not going to control you; you are going to control it. I could hardly say the words when it was happening because I was in denial. Cancer happens to other people, not me!

Truth is, everybody is always the other guy until they are the guy. Even being the guy, I still didn't believe I was the guy it was happening to, but I was, and it was, and this is what I did about it. Stay with me because you're going to be able to solve your little situation, laugh your ass off, cry a couple of times, and feel mighty and powerful throughout the entire process as you step out into the unknown, unknown and experience the prism of uncertainty.

Ready, set, let's go!

TROUBLE IN PARADISE

Here is how it all started for me.

Besides my children, one of my great passions is playing guitar for a contemporary praise and worship band at a local Lutheran church. One weekday, as I was working through the Sunday song list, holding the guitar close to my chest, as one does (and yes, I was playing naked guitar, which, funny as you might find it, actually saved my life), I felt moisture in the area of my breast. Later that morning, as I put the guitar up, and prepared to shower, I noticed a yellow substance dried on my flanks. My first thought was that Tommie, my son, had put water into my guitar for some strange reason, and it had leaked out onto me as I played. I showered, got dressed, and went to work, thinking nothing further about it. When I came home from work that evening, and was changing into my pajamas, I noticed fluid of the same color in my bra. What the...Oh, my God! My breast was leaking! The fluid was coming from me.

I told myself to keep it together, calmly get the children ready for bed, and investigate the matter further. My mind was racing, a thousand miles an hour, actually obsessing! What could this be? Too bad the physician's office isn't open at 11:00 pm, because I wanted to have my doctor paged right then and there. Because of my experience in the health care industry, I knew I had reason to be concerned. I tried to sleep that night, but worry wouldn't let me. I called my gynecologist first thing that morning, trying not to sound like a crazed lunatic, stressing the urgency of my findings, and my need to make an immediate appointment. Once I was examined at his office, he was calm; I was not. He gave me an order for a diagnostic mammogram with a follow-up ultrasound. I went to the imaging center straight away, and as they performed the diagnostic mammogram, the compression caused my breast to leak. At this point, I knew there was no denying that something was definitely wrong. After the mammogram, I underwent the ultrasound, and there appeared to be a papilloma, which is a benign tumor. I wasn't sure if what I saw was actually there, or perhaps I saw something I feared was there? The technician was concerned, and couldn't say anything, and went to get the radiologist. I tried to keep my composure while I waited for the radiologist to come in and complete the scan, then incurred more days of waiting for the final report.

To my astonishment, the report came back inconclusive, but with a recommendation for further testing, a ductogram. The report made no mention of what occurred when I was in the mammography suite at the imaging center, where my breast oozed yellow fluid. On top of that, the recommendation from my gynecologist upon reading the report was that I could come back in six months, for further evaluation of the breast at that time. Basically, if I didn't want to have a "situation/episode/

breast disease," I could come back in six months and we would reassess.

I walked out of that office fuming, unbelievable fear, and anger began to well up inside me. Something was seriously wrong, I just knew it, and I was not going to accept the findings of this report. A leaking breast is not a normal healthy breast for a woman of my age. I immediately scheduled an appointment with a breast surgeon with whom I was familiar with, and to whom I had referred several friends. She was gracious enough to get me in the next day.

It was at this point that I began to feel alone in this unfolding medical nightmare, and it was starting to suffocate me. I phoned my cousin Cindy, who lived nearby, and shared with her in as much detail as possible about what I was going through, all the while trying to dilute the severity of my concerns with my own brand of humor. I swore Cindy to complete and utter secrecy (our mothers are sisters), and I told her I was feeling out of control. She offered to go with me to the appointment the next day, and I was somewhat relieved to have someone to share this information with. I was making myself nuts under the strain of coping with the diagnosis I had already made in my mind, but which I had not yet formally received. We agreed to meet at my house the next morning.

As I approached the surgeon's office with Cindy that morning, I noticed under the surgeon's name on the door, that she specialized in diseases of the breast. I'm thinking, "What does that mean? Well, can we treat my breast disease with medicine?" "No," I tell myself, "She's a surgeon, Cathy—they open up the body with a scalpel!" I walked through the door and proceeded, with trepidation. The surgeon conducted an ultrasound, and confirmed that there was indeed a papilloma. We then discussed excision plus mammoplasty. I was disturbed by the findings but at the same time hugely relieved. At least now I could begin to move forward, or so, I thought.

After this diagnosis, I went to see two plastic surgeons, both very highly regarded, and one of them said the clusters on the right side felt like tumors. Until those were cleared, he wouldn't perform the surgery. I then made another appointment with the initial breast surgeon, and endured even more days of worry and fear leading up to that appointment. She performed a fine-needle aspiration, and the results came back: Atypia. As a follow-up, she ordered a breast magnetic resonance imaging study or Breast (MRI), which came back with benign findings. It all seemed pretty straightforward to me. We scheduled the surgery to remove the papilloma on the right side and then at my insistence, I scheduled the plastic surgeon to perform mammoplasty on both breasts immediately following. I was going to come out of this with gorgeous BMW breasts. I paid the plastic surgeon five thousand dollars out of my pocket; that was the portion of the surgery the insurance wouldn't cover because mammoplasty was considered cosmetic surgery by my insurance company. (Even later, when the findings came back as cancer, they would not reimburse me for the expenses because the plastic surgeon was out of network.) I didn't mind the out of pocket expense, as this surgeon was, and still is one of the best in Houston. Remember, I was going to have a whole new chassis at the end of this surgery, so I was both relieved and excited, and focused on the end result. I scheduled the surgery feeling confident and reassured.

In the interim, I traveled to California on a pre-planned trip for my grandmother's ninetieth birthday party, and to visit my family; my brother Steve and his wife, Nikki, their son, Preston, who was five years old then, and their one-week-old twins, Elle and Grafton. I also planned to visit my other brother, Tom, his wife, Libby; and their twins, Tommy and Molly. For a week, I forgot about my own situation and plunged head first into having a blast with my family, especially my nieces and nephews—they were a great distraction. My sister-in-law Nikki had been diagnosed with Stage IIB breast cancer, estrogen receptor (ER) negative, progesterone receptor (PR) negative and HER-2-positive, during her pregnancy, except for the little kids, things were topsy turvy during the visit.

Nikki's surgeon performed a lumpectomy while she was still pregnant with the twins, and her oncologist was waiting until she was three weeks postpartum to begin six rounds of chemotherapy, followed by radiation and a year of trastuzumab. I had arrived one week after the twins were born, to assist Nikki, and be an extra pair of hands. I had no intention of sharing my own encounter with breast disease, and what I was going through at the time. That week, I kept my diagnosis to myself, but all the while, I was obsessed about what awaited me when I got home. I decided to focus my energy on helping Nikki by offering support and understanding. I came to California armed with several books, lots of love, and motivation to help her see that this was not a death sentence, and that she would come out of this healthy, successful, alive, and thriving. Nikki was absolutely terrified at the time, and it was hard to console her. Little did I know, we would later be going through breast cancer treatment together.

I came back from California, and had an open and frank discussion with my nanny, Liseth—who, by the way is an absolute saint, and should be referred to as St. Liseth. She had everything together to tend to the children during my upcoming twenty three hour hospital stay. I was preparing myself mentally for the surgery, and despite my years of working in diagnostic imaging, it never occurred to me to check my own images or report before I went to surgery to confirm findings, recommendations, and the interpreting radiologist.

In hindsight, that was a huge oversight on my part, always review your reports once you receive them and keep a copy for your records. Check the signatures and verify that the radiologist who is interpreting your breast studies is the one you want to perform the service for you. I went to surgery that morning thinking about how unbelievably wonderful, and fun, the end result of this surgery would be. In just a few weeks' time, I would have smoking hot, perky, new breasts. I fell into a deep sleep on the operating table with images of myself in a Pamela Anderson style Baywatch swimsuit. Seven hours later, I awoke to the most unbelievable scenario I have ever experienced in my life to date.

My cousin Cindy, who planned to greet me after surgery, was sitting by my bed, along with my then estranged husband, we'll call him Zeus. I'm thinking, "Why is he here?" Unbeknownst to me, both Cindy and Zeus had been told of the findings postoperatively, and were both sitting in front of me, looking blanched. I was groggy and disoriented, but I remember thinking, "Success! Cindy looks like a ghost, because it's killing her that my new rack looks better than hers. Zeus is grief stricken because now I have an amazing, high and tight new rack he'll never see." I started to laugh, and then I snapped to the fact that the surgeon was speaking to them, explaining that they had found carcinoma, and are recommending a unilateral mastectomy. She was not looking at me, but was talking about me. I heard her say she had finished the excisions, and the plastic surgeon came in to commence the mammoplasty. Once the plastic surgeon had begun to form the base of the pedicle she found a tumor. She excised it, opened it up, and sent it to the lab, and the preliminary report came back as carcinoma. She decided to finish the surgery as we had agreed, not knowing what I would want to do next.

From my hospital bed, I couldn't believe what I was hearing and assumed they were wrong. I began correcting them, saying, "You mean a papilloma, right? Not carcinoma!" I was thinking they were all confused, because two of the three of us are not in the industry. I'm also hitting the morphine pump pretty hard because this is too weird for color TV, and the pain is becoming more acute as I am becoming more aware. I began vomiting and thinking I was high, and that this was all part of postoperative anesthesia. Except they were continuing to talk, and I was continuing to vomit while, at the same time, telling my support system, "Guys, don't worry! There's been a mix-up. I'll get it straightened out." I tried reassuring them that I was going to be very philosophical about this, that there had been a mistake. I told the surgeon to get a hold of a certain doctor to get things sorted out, and she said, "Will do."

After a while, Cindy, and Zeus left, and I was by myself, continuing to vomit and process this news, notice, this news, not, "my news." I didn't own any of this cancer business at this point. The surgeon came in later that night alone, and I ripped her a new one for having had that conversation with my cousin and the children's father without my consent, which by the way, is a huge Health Insurance Portability and Accountability Act (HIPAA) violation, except I didn't tell her this because I was too high, and sick from the morphine. I did however, have the presence of mind to realize I was going to need referrals. We got through all that, and I asked her to call the radiologist who I thought had read the MRI. She told me another radiologist did the interpretation, one who was not on faculty with the academic entity I thought was reading the breast MRI's—starting to see the picture, because I was.

As it turned out, the group I understood to be interpreting the breast imaging studies hadn't been reading for that breast center for about a year. They don't announce those little subcontractor switches either, so I didn't know that the highly respected breast imager I thought had read my breast studies was not the one currently reading at the breast center. Another breast imaging group had been subcontracted to provide the breast imaging portion of the service. Now the gravity and seriousness of the situation had taken hold, and I knew beyond a shadow of doubt there was serious trouble in my paradise. This was my new reality, and I had to work through it, but what was I going to do? Still, that night, I couldn't believe the scene, and as I slowly gained more and more clarity, I began reliving it continually and wondering, "What does this mean? Where do I start? What are the next steps to steer my way out of this?" I fell in and out of sleep all night worrying and wondering…crying and laughing… trying to stay positive while filling up with angst.

Twenty-three hours later, Cindy, who had just broken her foot, came up to my room in a wheelchair, pushing herself with one leg, and I was never so happy to see her! She was my ticket to get out of the hospital. I said, "You're my ride?" I am the eldest of the two, and I am forever assuming the caretaker, the mother, and mentor roles. Here I was, completely bandaged from the surgery, devastated by the most shocking news of my life, and less than twelve hours after my operation, I was pushing her out the doors of the hospital! Hilarious! I went home and waited for seven days to hear and review the final pathology report from the surgery.

In the interim, I was trying to recover, falling out of cars because prior to surgery, I had 44 FF breasts. Now I had gorgeous full C cup breasts, which I was thrilled with, but I had a little bit of a balance problem. I looked fabulous in and out of my clothes—a very important observation at this particular juncture! I was still thinking I could keep these gorgeous new girlfriends I had just spent a fortune on and I was determined to move forward.

Cancer Cat Advice:

∞∞∞

Once you begin to be worked up for breast disease, it is imperative that you keep all of your imaging and pathology reports. Know the location of your pathology specimens, should you want to send them to other institutes for additional opinions. Take The Cancer Cat's Clinical Consultation Worksheet, Anatomic Stage/Prognostic Groups which includes Cancer Staging Criteria and TNM Tables, and the Cancer Staging Summary Discussion Document. Take these and the other discussion documents with you, and keep them up to date as information is disclosed to you. This is your life; it is critical that you take responsibility for yourself, do your research, and remain informed throughout the entire process. You will live with the effect of each clinical decision, not anyone else, only you!

Remember two things; there should be no suffering and prevention should be in place always. Have your mammograms and reports explained to you in as much detail as you require to understand what they reveal and what it means for you. I worked in the industry, and it never occurred to me to check my own report or images before I went to surgery to verify the findings and check the signature of the interpreting radiologist. Besides, my findings were benign, so I had less reason to doubt. If only...Later I would learn that if had I reviewed the report, and verified the signatures, I might have saved myself some unnecessary surgery and pain.

∞∞∞

BREAST CANCER BOMB DROPPED

Seven days later, I went to see the plastic surgeon to have the gorgeous BMWs looked at and surgical wounds checked. Yes, I wanted to change my name to Your Gorgeousness! I had already ordered my red Pamela Anderson swimsuit and I was ready to get into it. I was escorted into the exam room with my cousin Cindy, and we waited an exceptionally long time (never a good sign!) before being seen. The plastic surgeon finally came in with a serious, all-business look; she was cautious, and holding the surgical pathology report, then said the three dreaded words nobody wants to hear, "You have cancer." Not only did I have cancer—I had it in eleven out of fourteen sections of the breast. There was a lot of ductal carcinoma in situ (DCIS) some invasive ductal carcinoma (IDC). Then she reiterated she would treat the wounds from this point on, and recommended that I go to a tertiary care facility immediately for further evaluation. I couldn't fathom what I was hearing! Cindy and I left in silence.

I was still on oral pain medication and not quite myself. When you hear DCIS, IDC, lobular carcinoma in situ (LCIS), invasive lobular carcinoma (ILC), inflammatory breast cancer (IBC), or tubular carcinoma (TC), it may as well be JKLM-NOP! You don't know or care at that moment what any of those letters stand for or how much there is of each in terms of millimeters or centimeters. Most patients don't understand a pathology report, the measurements and the significance they have on determining the treatment plan. They are processing the three dreaded words they just heard and considering the what-if's. Cindy was looking at me with the what's-next look, shocked herself. I blurted out, "I'm thinking, I'm thinking. I am thinking I need a paper bag because I am about to hyperventilate!" My problem was defined right there.

What was I thinking? I was so angry and disappointed because, well, now what the bleep do I do? I suddenly found myself in what is known as an uncertain decision space, looking through life from the prism of uncertainty and with a plethora of information to try to sift through. I couldn't really see the situation for what it was, let alone the outcome I actually desired.

What do you do in this situation? You cry, a lot! You might consider making it look like an accident, so the family collects the life insurance, and you don't have to go through this. You get second opinions on the third opinions and finally have to decide, okay what am I going to do? Still, it isn't clear, so now comes all the internet web queries, and all you see are statistics and you flip out.

Cancer Cat Tip:

∞∞∞

Never, and I mean never take a turn towards Negative Town. Everything you are going through at this moment is not permanent. Therefore, you need to focus your energy on all of the change management required to get yourself aligned with experts that can provide you with the information you need to put together your plan of care and quickly.

∞∞∞

Cancer Cat Advice:

∞∞

This is the point where you begin to put together your medical team, schedule all of your appointments, and consult with your specialists. I've provided example forms on the following 5 pages, but download and print the actual forms from my website here: http://www.thecancercat.com/forms.pdf to use. You need to track all of the information and data you are being given as you meet with surgeons, plastic surgeons, oncologists, and radiation oncologists. Once your case is presented to the tumor board, and you meet with each of your clinical specialists, you will need to take these discussion documents with you to all of your visits going forward to keep track of all of the information disclosed.

Please take a friend or trusted family member with you to provide assistance with writing down the information received. Make two copies of the forms, one for you and one for your scribe. You will want to go back and reevaluate the information disclosed at your consultations as well as all of the recommendations given to you for your treatment and plan of care.

∞∞

CANCER DIAGNOSIS CLINICAL CONSULTATION WORKSHEET
KEEP ALL IMAGING AND PATHOLOGY REPORTS

BIOPSY RESULTS	TUMOR GRADE
Ductal Carcinoma In Situ - DCIS	Type of Carcinoma
Invasive Ductal Carcinoma - IDC	Node Dissection – Yes or No
Lobular Carcinoma In Situ - LCIS	TUMOR FOCALITY
Invasive Lobular Carcinoma - ILC	Single Focus
Inflammatory Breast Cancer - IBC	Multi Foci – Number ( )
Medullary Carcinoma - MC	Tumor Size ( )
Tubular Carcinoma - TC	Grade
Any Other Designation Subtyping	Margins
1.	Lymph Node Sampling
2.	Sentinel Lymph Node
3.	Axillary Dissection
RECEPTORS	Lymph Node Status
Estrogen Receptor (ER) – Positive or Negative	RECONSTRUCTION
Progesterone Receptor (PR) – Positive or Negative	Immediate or Delayed Reconstruction
HER2 – Positive or Negative	Temporary Expanders
Other Ancillary Studies:	Permanent Implants
Ki-67 – Findings:	Free Flap Reconstruction
GRADE OF TUMOR	DIEP
1.	Latissimus Dorsi
2.	TRAM
3.	GAP
TUMOR STAGING	Expander Fill Procedures
Stage 0 – In Situ	Permanent Implant Exchange

	Other Reconstruction:
Stage IA	ADJUVANT CHEMOTHERAPY RECOMMENDED – YES OR NO
Stage IB	Type of Chemo:
Stage IIA	Number of Infusions:
Stage IIB	Infusion Start Date:
Stage IIIA	Infusion Completion Date:
Stage IIIB	Port Required – Yes or No
Stage IIIC	Port Insertion Date:
Stage IV	Port Removal Date:
NEOADJUVANT CHEMOTHERAPY RECOMMENDED	RADIATION THERAPY RECOMMENDED
Yes	Number of Treatments:
No	Number of Boosts:
PRE-SURGICAL RADIATION RECOMMENDED	Radiation Planning and Start Date:
Yes	Radiation and Boost Finish Date:
No	HORMONE SUPPRESSION AND ADJUVANT THERAPY RECOMMENDED
SURGICAL RECOMMENDATIONS	Tamoxifen
Lumpectomy	Anastrozole (ARIMIDEX®)
Partial Mastectomy	Other
Unilateral Mastectomy	Trastuzumab (Herceptin®) Recommended: Yes or No
Bilateral Mastectomies	Number of Infusions
RESECTION DATA	Start Date:
Number of Lymph Nodes Positive ( )	Completion Date:
Number of Lymph Nodes Examined ( )	

CANCER STAGING SUMMARY INFORMATION DISCUSSION DOCUMENT:
UTILIZE WITH CLINICAL CONSULTATION WORKSHEET

Changes in Staging	Review the table summarizing breast cancer staging and make sure your staging is complete
Anatomic Considerations - TNM	Primary Tumor Regional lymph nodes Metastatic sites
Rules for Classification	Clinical Pathologic
Prognostic Features	Identification and discussion of nonanatomic prognostic factors important in each disease reported
Definitions of TNM	T: Primary tumor N: Regional lymph nodes M: Distant metastases
Anatomic Stage/Prognostic Groups	
Prognostic Factors (Site-Specific Factors)	Required for staging Clinically significant
Grade	
Histopathologic Type	
Refer to the Staging Form	
Refer to the Clinical Consultation Worksheet	
Physician Name/Address	Clinical Comments

ANATOMIC STAGE/PROGNOSTIC GROUPS

STAGE	TUMOR	NODE	METASTASES
Stage 0	Tis	N0	M0
Stage 1A	T1[a]	N0	M0
Stage 1B	T0	N2mi	M0
Stage 1B	T1[a]	N1mi	M0
Stage IIA	T0	N1[b]	M0
Stage IIA	T1[a]	N1[b]	M0
Stage IIA	T2	N0	M0
Stage IIB	T2	N1	M0
Stage IIB	T3	N0	M0
Stage IIIA	T0	N2	M0
Stage IIIA	T1[a]	N2	M0
Stage IIIA	T2	N2	M0
Stage IIIA	T3	N1	M0
Stage IIIA	T3	N2	M0
Stage IIIB	T4	N0	M0
Stage IIIB	T4	N1	M0
Stage IIIB	T4	N2	M0
Stage IIIC	Any T	N3	M0
Stage IV	Any T	Any N	M1

aT1 includes T1mi.

bT0 and T1 tumors with nodal micro metastases only are excluded from Stage IIA and are classified Stage IB.

American Joint Committee on Cancer – 2010 7th edition

APPOINTMENT WORKSHEET

Physician Name	Specialty	Physical Address	Corre- sponding Hospital	Appoint- ment Date	Appoint- ment Time	Insurance In Network	Surgery Date	Chemo Infusion Date	Radiation Oncology Date

COMMUNICATION OF CANCER TO
FAMILY, FRIENDS, AND EMPLOYERS

Once you hear the word "cancer", you are at the very least, tortured and completely twisted up with multiple questions swirling around and co-mingling in your brain about how to begin navigating your way through this. Therefore, you should take all the time you need to put together a plan that you are comfortable with, and then communicate as you wish with family, friends and most especially employers.

My family, with the exception of my cousin Cindy, all live halfway across the country. My mother, Molly, whom I love and have the greatest respect for, are worlds apart on our views, politics, work preferences, you name it. When we get together or have a family gathering, it is a summit, everyone is very opinionated and outspoken. When I informed Mother of the cancer diagnosis, she interrupted me early in the conversation and literally pleaded with me not to tell her anymore because it was too much, terribly upsetting, and she just couldn't handle it. I couldn't believe what I was hearing. I responded by yelling, "I can't believe you don't want to hear about the most important, and difficult thing in my life! I am even more mortified than you are right now." She was crying and said, "This is too much, I can't bear it, and can't hear anymore, please stop!"

I knew I was going to need her support if I was going to get through this. I hung up the phone, sobbing uncontrollably. However, it didn't take very long before it occurred to me—this is what people are talking about when the "cat's out of the bag," some people can handle cancer, and some can't. Molly really couldn't handle Nikki and I having cancer at the same time, or anytime for that matter. It scared her to death, I could see that. I think she made the mental leap from the cancer diagnosis to my funeral, and it was just too much for her to bear. I decided no more cancer conversations or cancer chats with Molly.

In all fairness, I needed to give her time to digest the information and reach her own peace with it. Throughout my treatment and recovery, my mother was extremely supportive in so many ways. She took care of the nursing expense the week following the big surgery and many other precious things that made it a lot easier and more comfortable for the children and I. She called every day during chemo and radiation when it meant a lot to me, and I sincerely appreciated it. I got over the fact that she couldn't talk about what I was going through. Instead, I would share with her stories of other women and men I had met in the hospital and during treatment. I did meet fascinating men and women, too, and could tell you a million different stories of their treatment and recovery. Often, it baffled me how many people I met that didn't have any idea about what their treatment was doing to their bodies or what alternatives there might have been for them. Many of them never questioned their doctor's findings or recommendations. I was stunned by that which made me even more determined to record everything that was happening to me. I decided that I would share my experience, and the tools I was creating along the way to empower others to take charge, and partner with their physicians for a more deliberate and satisfying outcome.

Cancer Cat Tip:

Quick note, when the people you love can't be there in the capacity you want or intend for them to be, let it go and forgive them. They can still support you in their own way; you just need to give them permission to discover what that means for themselves, or tell them what would be most helpful for you. They can send money, pass along information and referrals, or assist you with other tasks such as cooking, cleaning or tending to your home, and children, if necessary.

All of my friends were very loving, supportive, and understanding. I didn't discuss much of what was going on with anyone outside of my close and proximal circle because there was too much turbulence occurring in my life at that time. I needed to play my cards close to my chest and proceeded that way through the various phases of my treatment.

Informing your employer is where it can become very difficult. You will want to make sure you have all the information before you initiate a cancer diagnosis conversation and the implementation of a treatment plan with your employer. You need to review your healthcare benefits, and whether cancer treatment is covered within your policy and what institutions are contracted with your insurer. Familiarize yourself and understand what your treatment options are and the location of your treatment institutions. You will want to prepare robust timelines from start to finish.

After you have educated yourself about your health care benefits and provider plan, I want to encourage you to thoroughly review your employer's policy for FMLA or Family Medical Leave Act. Your employer's Intermittent Family Medical Leave Act, the sick and vacation time and how it is accounted for. Human Resources can help you with this, and must maintain your anonymity before you have the dialogue with your immediate supervisor. You will mostly likely need surgery and recovery time. If chemotherapy is recommended; you may need to take a day off for each infusion, although there are infusion centers that offer 24/7/365 infusion scheduling. Make sure you look into the infusion center's hours of operation, so you can plan your time off. Radiation can be scheduled early in the morning or late in the afternoon, but this may cause you to have to take unplanned time off. You may need an hour or more daily depending on the location of your radiation treatment center, so understand the time off policy and account for any unpaid leave that you may encounter. This is an unintended consequence of cancer treatment if not properly planned for, and trust me, cancer is always unplanned!

The health care organization I worked for at the time of my diagnosis was decent. However, my supervisor was not very keen on any of this cancer business (but who could blame her, neither was I). She had brought me up from the Department of Diagnostic and Interventional Imaging, just months prior to my diagnosis, and must have been thinking she got a lemon once I informed her about what was happening to me. You see, for some employers, their management team may not realize that twenty five percent of their workforce will be affected with a degenerative disease during their working career. It is prudent for everyone—employers and employees—to know how to handle all phases of cancer treatment planning for their employees. Again, what I discovered is that everybody is always the other guy until they are the guy, then it's all different because they are enlightened! If you get one who has been the guy, you're good. Sadly, I didn't; she was the other guy, and didn't advocate for my time or projects, etc. — Very disheartening.

Cancer Cat Advice:

Make sure all of your cancer staging is complete before you make any decisions, particularly about surgical matters. Take all of the worksheets with you before you select a surgical strategy and treatment plan. Review your health care benefits to ensure your coverage is intact, and the facilities that offer the expertise you require are contracted with your insurance plan. Review the vacation, sick, paid time off policy and unpaid time off policy your employer utilizes and account for any differences financially to the best of your ability. Stop all bank drafts out of your checking accounts if you're going to need cash, and organize your finances so you can manage adding cancer treatment and costs in a probably already cramped budget. Bottom line, you need to get started with your treatment, sooner as opposed to later, so once you have gotten everything in place, inform your employer.

SCIENTIFIC METHODOLOGY
UTILIZING LEAN SIX SIGMA

I found this methodology to be very effective. Let's first discuss the goals and techniques utilized in Six Sigma, specifically DMAIC and how it can be utilized for problem solving by providing structure to what might have otherwise been chaos. Six Sigma aims to eliminate process variation and make process improvements based on the customer—you—with a definition of quality, and by measuring process performance and process change effects to implement a workable solution that can sustain the gains.

The Six Sigma technique I will discuss and utilize here is the 5-step DMAIC process:

— <u>D</u>efine the problem

— <u>M</u>easure the extent of the current situation

— <u>A</u>nalyze for root cause

— <u>I</u>mprove and implement a process plan effectively

— <u>C</u>ontrol the process to maintain the gain

DEFINE

Okay, you've heard the three dreaded words and now you're swirling around an Alice in Wonderland's Black Hole, thinking who's going to throw you a flare? I am—that's who!

As I previously mentioned, I was a former Director of Diagnostic and Interventional Imaging, and my very own mammography readings were incorrect. I went to surgery the first time for ductal excisions followed by mammoplasty, only to discover a tumor at the base of the pedicle and DCIS/IDC in eleven out of fourteen areas of the breast. I woke up thinking I had these beautifully sculpted BMW breasts only to find out I had breast cancer and needed a unilateral mastectomy right away. The most pressing question for me to address was what was I going to do about the other breast, if anything, and could I do immediate reconstruction? I was not thinking about chemotherapy or radiation; it gets more intense as we go. At that point, I still didn't know the magnitude of the problem, and didn't have a clue where to start, so I did the logical next step and backtracked into what happened.

I went to meet with a renowned tertiary care radiologist who I thought read the breast MRIs, who pointed out in no uncertain terms that it was there on the MRI's, that it was overlooked. In my naivety I assumed he was reading the images, in my false confidence I did not personally look at them. Had I done so, I would have seen what he later pointed out because I am in the industry and would have recognized it. Your question right now is most likely, "Cat, did you seek legal remedy?" No, I did not. There is tort reform in Texas, and the payout would have been miniscule for the time invested, and I had no desire to relive it and devote any of my time to that. There was no solution in filing suit against the breast imager, so it wasn't even contemplated. I decided to record everything in a logarithmic approach to maximize my outcome and nonrecurrence. If it worked, and it did, I would make it available to anyone seeking a solution to a breast cancer diagnosis and treatment. For me that was a much better use of my time and resources.

In the meantime, I had these beautiful, luscious breasts, and a couple of my dear friends, we'll call them Mr. and Mrs. Woods, had stopped by the house to check on me after the first surgery. It was about four weeks after the mammoplasty, and I was feeling good and looking great. I was talking about my breast reconstruction plans, and I unbuttoned my blouse and started to show them the approaches and what it would look like when completed. Mr. Woods said, "Cathy, please stop! Do you know how many years I have wanted to look at and grab your breasts? For years—my wife can attest to this," as his wife nodded affirmatively, confirming this fact about her husband, and my dear friend. "Give me a moment to gaze at all of this magnificence in front of me and let me tell you, they are incredible, and I love them. They were unbelievable before, but what can I say, you have made me a very happy man today!" I said, "You sand bag-ging S.O.B., you!" Then I rolled over on the couch, cracking up laughing as I always do when they come over.

The next day, it was back to the Internet to look at pictures of breast reconstructions while setting up appointments with all the respected oncologists, breast surgeons, and plastic surgeons here in Houston as well as outside of Texas. I was considering flying to other parts of the country because now I had a problem: my skin and blood supply had been compromised because of the prior surgery. A sentinel node biopsy was not done at the time of the first surgery because there was no knowledge of cancer in the first place, or the mammoplasty would not have been done. It would have been an excisional biopsy, and my options would have been different.

I had recovered enough from the first surgery and returned to work after seven working days off, looking and feeling great physically, but now had to put together my new medical team to partner with for the cancer treatment plan.

The large Houston health care system I worked for as a Lean Six Sigma Black Belt had some unbelievable talent onboard. We called ourselves the Super Hero Team. I was El Diablo; and there was Smokin' Hot; Cash; The Magic Man; and our boss, the Commander. There were two others, the Evil Twins, who worked in the Department of Diagnostic and Interventional Imaging. For the first time in my career, I had the privilege of working and being surrounded by colleagues who possessed remarkable intellect, great character, and all gathered in one small quarter of a hospital tower. After being adrift with all of the cancer conversations, being back at work reminded me, "You are a Black Belt, you cut data, and construct workflow process maps all day long. You can make tables, and maps do all sorts of miraculous things, reflect data and workflows in all sorts of ways, and groups are all different." What was needed were some power tools, a process map, a workflow and discussion documents to start navigating my way through this. I looked everywhere for information and found a lot of nutritional, spiritual, and self-help information but alarmingly little on strategy, and how to begin to navigate the health care maze with the added complexity of a breast cancer diagnosis.

I visited the Susan Komen message board, which was great. (Girls, special thanks to each and every one of you who divulged so much of your personal and medical information to me during that time. You gave me a lot of cyber encouragement, and I will be eternally grateful to each and every one of you all the days of my life. Update: This Cancer Cat is thriving and having a good time!) I visited it frequently at the time, and talked to other Komen Sisters who had a breast cancer experience, but I began to find out that each one was unique, or "N of 1," in that each breast cancer experience and treatment plan was as unique as the individual and the outcome.

This is what is called Define, or the D phase, defining the magnitude of the problem and writing your problem statement. Mine was, I have DCIS/IDC and will gain every piece of information available to make a viable treatment plan to save my life, and reduce the opportunities for recurrence and have beautiful breasts.

DEFINE

- » Prepare your problem statement.
- » Define the type of breast disease that you have.
- » Determine location of the breast centers and expertise you will consult with to determine your treatment plan.
- » Schedule appointments with the medical team to discuss treatment options.
- » Print out all of the Cancer Cat forms and discussion documents so you can evaluate the data as it becomes available to you: http://www.thecancercat.com/forms.pdf

<u>M</u>EASURE

I was exhausted from the news of the first surgery and diagnosis, but wasn't ready to throw in the towel and accept a cosmesis or a treatment plan I didn't want. My little peeps, Stephie and Tommie whom I refer to as my Chili's, were in my corner and needed me to keep it together. I decided to continue and began the next phase, called <u>M</u>easure.

Your tumor(s) and extent of the infiltrated area will need to be measured with a high level of precision. I suggest you have it measured by more than one entity and compare the pathology reports. You are asking the pathologists to measure the specimens in order to fully understand the extent of the disease, and for two reasons: (1) so that you will be accurately staged; (2) so you and your surgeon, oncologist, radiation oncologist and plastic surgeon can partner to create a solution that meets your requirements. I have included the stages of breast cancer in the Anatomic Stage and Prognostic Groups for you to review. I also want to encourage you to visit the National Cancer Institute's website for greater understanding:

WWW.CANCER.GOV

I sent my pathology specimens and slides to three different

pathology labs for evaluation, and in the end they were all pretty close. I had consults with all three different entities, discussing the various approaches, surgical strategies, and treatment plans. I couldn't really make a decision at that point, because I didn't have complete information regarding the results that the big surgery would yield.

My tolerance was going south—so south, in fact that while I was sitting at a renowned cancer institute, waiting for another consult absolutely, steaming and two seconds from sliding down the escalator head first,—picture this—with smoke coming out of my face, and turning red at the same time? Yes, all of that was what I was feeling, when this woman whom I had never seen before, and didn't know from Adam, and to this day don't know, said to me, "Do you know how to stay in the moment?" Her question took me completely by surprise and threw me off guard.

I replied, "If I knew that, do you think I would be sitting here pacing and looking berserk? Besides, I hate those metaphors. I do not like to hear, 'Take it easy,' 'One day at a time!' I think those sayings are worthless and never deliver one result."

"That is not the question," she said. "Do you know how to stay in the moment?"

I said, "Obviously, I don't, or I wouldn't sound like this." I then asked her, "OK, tell me, how do you stay in the moment?"

She said, "What happens to you when you go to the past?"

"I have regrets."

"That's right!" she said. "What happens to you when you go to the future?"

The tears are rolling down my face now, and I said, "I just get so anxious and feel out of control when I go to the future."

She sat down next to me and put her hand on my leg and said, "That's right! What happens to you right here, right now, you and me?"

"I'm okay," I answered.

She said, "That's right; that is how you stay in the moment."

It felt like I was in the presence of an angel for those few minutes. Then I heard my name called and off I went for my appointment, and I never saw her again. That advice has remained with me from that day forward, and today when I come unglued, and believe me, I can come unglued, it is because I get ahead of the right here, right now. That woman saved my sanity by sharing simple but sound advice, and now I am passing that pearl of wisdom onto you. It holds me steadfast when I am facing the prism of uncertainty, and keeps the moment so much sexier.

Now, you have received all of your measurements from your pathology and you have them recorded. I had Stage IIA breast cancer. The staging could have changed at the time of my second surgery; node involvement was unknown at the first surgery. However, the findings of the second surgery didn't affect the staging, (although it can). I had Stage IIA and continued to have Stage IIA even after the bilateral mastectomies and reconstruction.

The Measure phase or M portion of your discovery won't take long, but it may take some time before you receive all of the pathology reports back from your various entities and compare them against one another. You will need to continue to set up your appointments in the interim. Let's get ready to Analyze our Defined problem and Measurements that will determine the cancer staging and its implications on a viable treatment plan.

MEASURE

Once you have received and collected all the data from your specimen measurements, you will need to understand the following on your pathology report for the Measure phase:

- » Tumor size
- » Staging
- » Number of positive nodes
- » Hormone receptors
- » Tumor grade
- » K i–67

Take the Clinical Consultation Worksheet and all other Cancer Cat forms and discussion documents with you to all clinical visits and log all the information received from your pathology reports as well as your medical team's advice and counsel. Plan on archiving all of your pathology reports, imaging reports, and clinical consultation information, and keep all of your consultation forms updated as new data is received.

Cancer Cat Tip:

◇◇◇

Before you get started with this portion of your planning, go and get yourself a mood ring. That way, your loved ones, depending on the color of your ring, will know whether to move in—because the color suggests you are loving and affectionate or back off—because your homicidal tendencies are surfacing. I solved most of the mood swings and the fallout with family, friends, and work with a pretty little mood ring from the local dollar store!

◇◇◇

<u>A</u>NALYZE

During the <u>A</u>nalyze phase, you will begin to review all of the data and start to assign scores to the treatment options discussed. It is now critical that you understand each therapy's numeric as it relates to nonrecurrence and assign the appropriate score within your matrix. With a breast cancer diagnosis, the <u>A</u>nalyze phase generally begins when you consult with your oncologist(s), it can also be with your other medical team members, but as a rule it is with your oncologist. If you are not a statistics person, which most are not, it can become "sadistics" because you now have to make life threatening and life-saving decisions based on probabilities with therapies and outcomes changing continually. If this is not your specialty, take someone with you. I have prepared several worksheets you can take with you that are located within the book. Copy them, or tear them out, but whatever you do, please utilize and modify them as you wish to make sure you have all the information you need.

There are several matrices one can utilize to determine their final choice and review concerns associated with any Improvement solution or implementation plan. I utilized a criteria decision matrix which is placed here for you to objectively weigh the options, and will assist you with the decision making you will need to make once every treatment option or alternative has been presented and discussed with you.

CRITERIA DECISION SOLUTION MATRIX

Improvement	Solution Example	Solution 1	Solution 2	Solution 3	Solution 4	Solution 5	Solution 6	Solution 7
Surgery	70							
Immediate Reconstruction	Proceed							
Delayed Reconstruction	N/A							
Neoadjuvant Chemotherapy								
Adjuvant Chemotherapy	4							
Neoadjuvant Radiation								
Adjuvant Radiation	3							
Hormone Suppression	17							
Trastuzumab (Herceptin®)	N/A							
Other Adjuvant Therapies								
Total Percent Probability of Nonrecurrence	95%							
Total Score	10							

The matrix above will assist you with selecting your solution for your cancer treatment, depending on what is critical to quality for you. Prior to a treatment plan selection, review the weighted percentage provided to you for each therapy and its weight toward nonrecurrence. Consider each therapy or combination of therapies you may benefit from, then calculate the sum in the Total Percent Probability of Nonrecurrence. Score each solution and the impact it will have on your outcome and make your decision. Utilize a one to ten scoring system, with one being lowest, and ten the highest.

For those of you who don't have the luxury of taking someone with you, a recording device is helpful so you can replay the conversations, and place the information you have received where it belongs if you don't have a scribe. Trust me, your mind is going a thousand miles an hour, and if you're the one asking the questions, and writing down the answers, you can make mistakes. Have a recording device or another person with you that is competent during any of your clinical consultations, particularly when you are speaking with your oncologist. I have included immediate and delayed reconstruction within the Cancer Diagnosis Clinical Consultation Worksheet for you to utilize when you are meeting with your specialists. There is significantly more detail that your physicians will review and discuss with you in greater depth. Treatment plans can affect reconstruction plans, and this will need to be considered and factored into your criteria and decision matrix. There were requirements and preferences I had in terms of what was critical to quality for me. You will be uniquely different in terms of what is a critical requirement or element for you or a preference for you, as you consider all of your options. Requirements are not negotiable; preferences are, so you will need to determine what those are for yourself.

BREAST CANCER TREATMENT
SELECTIONS: FIVE SCENARIOS

I was back on the Internet and hitting every search engine, trying to find out some obscure cure beside surgery, chemo, and radiation or a clinical trial that would offer me something other than surgery, chemo and radiation, and thinking, what do I do? I came to the conclusion there are really only five scenarios to consider. There are subsets, but primarily these five.

Here are the five breast cancer treatment scenarios that most patients will fall into, without reconstruction discussed here. These are very generalized, and I want to encourage you to consult with your physician experts for specificity and greater detail.

SCENARIO 1:

Do nothing!:

Go home and live your life as though there was no cancer diagnosis. Some people opt to take care of it themselves with alternative approaches. Caution, you won't get any support from your formally trained medical clinicians regarding that decision if a treatment scenario is recommended, so beware.

Scenario 2:

Surgery:

You are a surgical patient. You have the tumor excised, all of the margins are clear, you have no nodal involvement, and depending on the receptors, you will receive hormone suppression therapy if indicated and follow-up visits.

Scenario 3:

Surgery and Radiation:

You have a lumpectomy, unilateral or bilateral mastectomies and will have radiation to ensure that any remaining cells are radiated. Hormone suppression if indicated and follow-up visits.

Scenario 4:

Surgery and Chemo:

You have a lumpectomy or unilateral mastectomy or bilateral mastectomies, and it has been determined that you will benefit from either neoadjuvant or adjuvant chemotherapy. Neoadjuvant is chemotherapy given before surgery, adjuvant chemotherapy is after. There are several different regimens and combinations of chemotherapy. Make sure you have familiarized yourself with the risks and benefits and possible side effects and discuss them with your oncologist to make sure there is a plan to mitigate any potential side effects during your treatment plan. Hormone suppression if indicated and follow-up visits.

I did adjuvant chemotherapy, and the infusions I received were docetaxel (Taxotere®) and cyclophosphamide (Cytoxan).

They were scheduled every three weeks on four separate infusion dates. Everything was very well managed. I never suffered and continued to work through the entire treatment phase.

SCENARIO 5:

Surgery, Chemo and Radiation:

You will have surgery followed by immediate reconstruction or delayed reconstruction or no reconstruction. Then, within 6-12 weeks post-op if you are receiving adjuvant chemotherapy, you will start your chemotherapy infusions, and radiation will follow. I want to point out that pre-surgical radiation may be ordered. Hormone suppression if indicated and follow-up visits.

ANALYZE

During the Analyze phase, you will need to investigate the tumor markers and verify your staging with your oncologist. Once you have examined the data and discussed the findings with your medical team, you will determine the approaches you will implement to eliminate the cancer.

» Know the specificity of the problem you are trying to solve for.

» Measure is vital, as is Analyze, so you can select a treatment scenario.

» Analyze all of the data given to you and look at the variable relationships to assist you with decision making.

» The Criteria Decision Matrix is useful as you review all of the alternatives and weigh your decisions on the probabilities for nonrecurrence.

» Archive all data from your pathology reports and your clinical consultations; keep all discussion documents and forms updated.
» Where does the data lead you?
» Get ready for Improve!

Note: You will retrieve this data from your pathology reports and your clinical consultations; keep all forms updated.

Cancer Cat Advice:

It is critical that you know and understand your TNM: Tumor status, Node status, and whether there are any Metastases, this is referred to as TNM. Utilize the Anatomic Stage and Prognostic Group Worksheet, to assist you with staging and TNM status. Remember, when it comes to chemotherapy recommendations and other forms of neo-adjuvant or adjuvant treatments, you will not receive a definitive or conclusive answer but a statistical probability for multiple scenarios. "If you do this, then this percentage; if you do that, then that percentage for nonrecurrence."

As you receive all of the information, you can begin to calculate where you will fall depending on the current meta-analysis. Your subspecialty expert, surgeon, oncologist or radiation oncologist will assist you with the interpretation of that statistical information, generally it will be your oncologist. Then you will be able to make calculated decisions, and the probability of you getting to the finish line is excellent.

ONCOLOGICAL CLINICAL
CONSULTATION: PRE-SURGERY

From the very beginning it was scenario two for me. I went in for bilateral mastectomies with immediate latissimus dorsi free-flap reconstruction. Postoperatively, it morphed into scenario four, and ultimately scenario five, so I had to redo my plan. For now, scenario two, which was surgery only and immediate free-flap reconstruction, and depending on what followed post operatively, chemo may be recommended per my pre-surgical follow-up visit with the oncologist and the breast surgeon.

Remember, I had been to the other cancer center and had follow-up ultrasounds to look at the breast and the nodes, and it showed no macro nodal involvement. I was deliriously happy upon hearing this result: It was the first A+ news I had received up to that point. I went back to the other breast cancer institute for an additional clinical consultation with my oncologist, who pointed out that I was not made aware that there may be micro involvement. The oncologist explained the difference between macro/micro nodal involvement and what it could mean for me. He then stated during the final pre-surgical visit that he would most likely recommend chemo because of how much DCIS/

IDC was present regardless of nodal involvement. Once adjuvant chemo was discussed, I froze and started to go in a tailspin, going a thousand miles an hour again, because this wasn't in the original plan. This was the first discussion of chemotherapy; I hadn't integrated the word into my vocabulary or treatment plan up to this point.

The first question I asked upon hearing the word chemotherapy was, "Will my hair fall out?" and the oncologist replied without hesitation, "Yes, it will." I was alone in a patient consultation room as he was telling me this, terrified, as most people are from hearing stories of former patients' and friends' side effects from chemotherapy that weren't mitigated. I was thinking about my children and what was going to happen to them.

Then I started going down in a vertical, firing off a series of questions like, "My net worth is X, how I will provide for the children if I become debilitated and can't work? If I die, they will cash out with X, should I make it look like an accident and hasten the inevitable…" The oncologist was listening to me and acted as though he was as cool as a cucumber. He had obviously heard these ramblings before and said, "Wait right here. I am going to get somebody for you to talk too." I felt like Freddie Kruger, wanting to use razor blades on the walls of that room, and in walked the manager of the infusion center, a cancer survivor herself with a cup of coffee in her hand. She introduced herself, sat down next to me, and said, "Wow, you look pretty together."

I said, "I've had a moment."

She said with a smile, "Continue to remain, calm." She then began to reiterate the following: "I did it all too. I had a lumpectomy, chemo, and radiation. I kept working, was tired, my hair fell out, but it is all back—as you can see—and that was a year ago. You can do this." She looked really put together, but was this the truth or fiction? Again, prior to this appointment, I had just come from the other renowned cancer center in the area who said no nodal involvement, so I was thinking no chemo. Needless to say, I was deeply concerned and disturbed.

I left the medical center, drove home, called my cousin in route, and conveyed to her what I had just been told. She was alarmed. In a moment of madness, I asked, "Do I go off a bridge, or run into a train, or something, and make it look like an accident?"

She said, "Of course, not! Don't do that."

With tears welling up in my eyes, I asked, "Why not? You're not the one who is going to fall off a cancer cliff!"

"Listen up," she said, "I went out of my way today and bought you a bunch of presents!"

"Presents?"

"Yes, presents—awesome presents, and all of your favorites too!"

"Seriously, or are you just saying this, so I won't do something drastic?" I grilled her.

She launched into the fact that I was behaving like absolute trash even questioning her integrity about buying the presents and having them for me. I forgot about my predicament because now I wanted her to e-mail me the receipts to confirm that there were indeed presents waiting for me in a couple of minutes. I love presents—they are even better than mood rings!

Cindy and I laughed hysterically, and as I got ready to cross the railroad tracks on the way to my residence—the same tracks I have traveled across daily for over twenty years…the tracks where I always look both ways and check the gates for my own piece of mind…, I didn't this time—you can understand why not at this particular moment. I proceeded to go across, and guess what? Yes, there was a train about nine yards from the driver's side of my vehicle. The conductor was blowing the horn and making a hand gesture at me. I just hit the accelerator in my Chevrolet Avalanche like I was a monster truck and drove right through with everything I had. I couldn't believe it…why today? Why now? That was one of many wake-up calls to alert me that I wanted to live, it also reminded me how much I really loved my life, and needed to get to work.

I finished the final consultations with the surgeon and plastic surgeon that would be performing the immediate reconstruction, and scheduled everything for August 1, 2007, thinking I can do this, no problem. At the time, I thought I could handle all this. I'll be in the hospital for four days, out and about right after that…I am about to share with you, closed captioned for the reality impaired. You cannot undergo this type of surgery without an advocate or someone with you, period! This was another serious misrepresentation I had at the time.

Prior to the big surgery, my brother Tom had phoned me from California to check in. It was about a week before the bilateral mastectomies and free-flap surgery date. Bless his heart, he offered to send his wife Libby out to care for me the week of the surgery. I declined in the interest of my twin niece and nephew because I couldn't see them starving to death while their mother was tending to me, which was an epic mistake on my part. I didn't have any idea as to the degree or magnitude of a free-flap reconstruction, or that I might need someone to advocate for me while I was undergoing a major surgery such as this one. My cousin was out of the country at the time for an extended period and couldn't be there with me, so I thought I would manage it on my own.

Do not think for a moment you can do this alone; this is very intricate, complex surgery, and you will need assistance. You simply cannot do this by yourself or have someone dropping by sporadically to check in on you for a few brief moments. This is beyond your scope and bandwidth to handle postoperatively, trust me. You will need someone who knows you—someone who is patient, persistent, accommodating, and understanding and who can stay with you in shifts and speak with your physicians should there be any issues. Hindsight being 100%, I instinctively knew my brother was, and is a fabulous father, and that he and the children would have been fine eating pizza, and fish sticks, or whatever he prepared for them. The twins would have been deliriously happy riding their tricycles throughout the house until their mother returned.

Cancer Cat Advice:

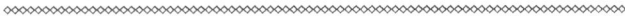

Set up your support system prior to your surgery. You will need assistance during your hospital stay and postoperatively with all tasks. Bathing, drain management, pain medication, care of young children, and any other chores you are responsible for until you are recovered enough to take them on again. If you don't have anyone to assist, or support is limited, contact Cancare or alternative organizations that can provide support via trained volunteers.

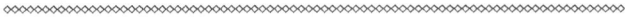

IMPROVE OR IMPLEMENTATION

The tumor(s) have been measured, and you have <u>A</u>nalyzed the risks and benefits of each scenario and treatment plan. Now you are ready to prepare a plan that you will implement for the Improve phase. For me, I would have bilateral mastectomies with immediate latissimus dorsi reconstruction, depending on the nodal involvement; chemo may or may not be recommended but most likely would.

How do you implement an Improve plan of action for breast cancer? You start by selecting a plan where the risks and benefits have been thoroughly evaluated. One that ultimately yields the maximal outcome, accommodates your critical to quality requirements, and allows you and your medical team the ability to execute it. I utilized scientific methodology, a superior power tool, (specifically DMAIC), and then organized a world-class team to provide the thorough subject matter expertise needed to implement such a plan. This is the part where you will need to draw on every bit of chutzpa you possess. Don't worry about what people think or how you come across. I want to remind you: At no time do you hesitate for one second or feel like you are being inappropriate with any question or request. It is your life and your body.

You will most likely need to partner with the following experts on your medical team:

Surgeon: Has to be great with a scalpel, and the best there is within your academic tertiary care community.

Oncologist: One who is great with chemotherapy and all other therapies. One who will discuss with you the probabilities of what each regimen will do, and reduce the likelihood of recurrence. Remember, write it all down and do your own research or have a member of your support team do this with— or for—you because you are responsible for the aftermath of every clinical decision and treatment you consent to. Calculate every decision wisely and make sure your staging is complete.

Plastic Surgeon: One who is great with a laser, suturing, gluing and will make you look hot! Not balanced in your clothes, but hot when you're walking out of the shower or any other place you like to visit naked. I want to encourage you to look at pictures of breast reconstructions, especially the type you are considering. Take some front and back anatomical human body drawings with you, and have the surgical lines drawn for you, so you can see where the scars will be. Talk with other people who have done the type of reconstruction you are considering. Consider visiting a breast cancer support group to talk and meet with others who have been through this. I will take my top off for anyone, and other wonderful women did it for me when I was curious about outcomes. Little sidebar, I also vote the newbie's breasts the best as *numero uno when I have been invited to parties where someone was about to undergo surgery, and wanted to know what the finished product looked like—my "silicone is a commodity"!*

Radiation Oncologist: You're going to receive a radiation burn of the century to your breast(s), so you need someone who understands radiation therapy and physics. A radiation oncologist who will execute safe and superior radiation planning and treatment. You will need to watch what happens to your skin in the process, and inform your radiation oncologist of any blistering or burning.

IMPROVE

» Create your solutions for improvement and implementation.

» Review the Decision Criteria Matrix created in Analyze, which will weigh relative importance to the values being disclosed regarding nonreccurrence.

» What scenario have you chosen to implement?

» What changes did you make to the original plan?

» How will you implement your plan and which medical experts will you partner with?

» Review before and after results of immediate or delayed reconstruction to determine whether you need to plan for this.

» Analyze all of the critical elements for nonreccurrence and your cosmesis before you make a final decision.

Cancer Cat's Advice:

Adjunct to the medical team but equally important is your Up Close and Personal Posse. You will determine who is on this team, and each member is tasked with a job. To have food prepared; to make sure your medicines are there, laid out and given to you on schedule; to provide assistance with the management of your drains, which will need to be emptied and accounted for until you can do this yourself. You will need someone to go with you to appointments or chemotherapy possibly. To sit with you, drive you, take care of you or your kids if need be, or clean your house until you are sufficiently recovered to perform all of those tasks. Liseth did ninety percent of everything on this list for me, and I am grateful beyond words. Check out Kris Carr's book Crazy, Sexy Cancer Tips. Carr spends a lot of time on the Posse. Very Important, and something I benefited from after reading her book.

SURGERY

I went to surgery August 1, 2007, and had a very complex case. I had consented to bilateral mastectomies with immediate free-flap latissimus dorsi reconstruction. What was supposed to be a seven-to-eight-hour surgery turned out to be a twelve hour surgery. I woke up around midnight, hearing the children's father and my plastic surgeon's voice. They both left, and I went back to sleep, but the pain pump was not set to continue to dose whether I'm asleep or not; it was set to deliver the drug with a manual hit of the pump for a dose. I woke up again at about three o'clock writhing in pain. A couple of nurses came in and worked feverishly to get it reset and make me comfortable, and I was horrible to them. Thank God, they kept working, but I had to get my soul back after the lashing I gave all of them. This is just one example of where having someone there with me would have been beneficial. They would have seen my agitation immediately and gotten help, and the pump would have been checked immediately and my pain managed. I drifted for days between unbearable pain and sleep.

A few days later, the attending surgeon's fellow entered my room and introduced himself, stating he was rounding for the attending. I mustered every bit of strength I had and said, "Wow, what a good looking fellow you are." He was so flattered, he blushed. Little did I know, he was about to drop another bomb on me by saying, "Oh by the way, there was nodal involvement, out of fifteen nodes, one was positive; that there were three micromets on the sentinel node affected." Had I known what he was going to blurt out, I would have taken back my comment. I said, "That confirms chemo, right?"

He said, "You will need to talk to the oncologist about that." Then he left the room abruptly. They always do that instead of hanging out while you process the gut-wrenching news.

Now I was thinking, good night, what else can go wrong? I can't feed myself, the pain meds hadn't been working properly, they were bolusing intravenous medications, and I am hallucinating at this point. This was another moment where I'm certain I was high—just high and this is all a mistake, but there was no mistake, and I knew I was in trouble. You can't give a person like me those types of medications without food intake, or an advocate to observe, feed, and tend to me, etc., and not expect to have things happen.

I will never forget the one night when I was lying there, literally considering wiping out the stupidity on the seventeenth floor of the hospital I was staying at. I learned several valuable lessons from a clinician's perspective. I always thought a person under the influence of intravenous drugs could control his or her actions. What I learned from my own experience of being on the other side of the bedrail, and not having enough strength to inch myself up in my bed with my feet, is that your dominant or rationale mind becomes the dormant mind, and the carnal mind becomes the dominant mind. All carnal mind wants is to be satiated and pain free and have anything else it desires. It has no sense of good or evil, correct or incorrect behaviors, and doesn't give a hoot about the cost to another individual. I was having conversations with a stage coach driver named Jedidiah who was in a picture hanging on the wall of my hospital room. We actually communicated for a couple of days. I was belligerent, furious, in agony, and had no one who could observe me, and state that something was seriously wrong. As it was, my children's father came up to the hospital when he could, which was sporadic, but he didn't understand any of what was happening to me, or what followed, and hence was not helpful.

In Zeus's defense, this was not his job. His role was to take care of our children. That he could and did do very well. With his limited interest and medical knowledge, other issues followed over my seven-day hospital stay. Again, I can't stress this enough, you must have an advocate who knows you and can let your surgeons know when the pain medicines are not working or pumps have disconnected; lines are fractured and need to be rescued because your behaviors are not normal; or you simply need a drink of water, food, or anything else you may desire or want assistance with.

It was now day four, and I am not home or anywhere close

to being ready to come home. Liseth could tell by watching the kid's dad that something was seriously wrong. She asked a lot of questions, and Zeus responded with my not being very responsive. Mostly out of it, dangerously high on a lot of intravenous pain medications, and behaving like something he had never seen before. Liseth knows me better than I know myself. She knows every day of my life, I wake up feeling like I'm seventeen years old and act like it most of the time—very high energy and nothing keeps me down—and knew that I would have been home by now. The narcotic thing was what had her worried, and from what she was hearing, it sounded like incomprehensible fear had set in. It had. I couldn't believe what was happening; I had always been in control, always up, mobile and running around and carrying on. Now at this point postoperatively, I couldn't inch myself up using my feet.

There is only one thing that can motivate me, and she knows what it is—the children. They're everything to me. It was summertime and everybody was out of school, so she gathered them up and readied the actual breakthrough for me. She cut out three little pictures of the children, Stephie, Tommie, and Joey, who is her son, and put them in a little stand that holds photo clips. It was my beautiful daughter in her bathing suit and hula skirt with her flower lei around her neck from her pool birthday party the year before. My son, Tommie, in his Superman costume, and her little son in his Superman costume, eating a lollipop. My daughter made me a queens crown with a handmade card, and Liseth put everything in a bag and sent it up with Zeus.

When he came to the hospital with that bag, I couldn't move, and for whatever reason Zeus thought if he angered me, I would be motivated to snap out of this "depression" he was certain was the cause of my behavior. He then got right up two inches from my blistered face—I am totally allergic to surgical tape—and started screaming at me with a nuclear capability to stop all of this nonsense and get it together. I couldn't rise, levitate, or perform as he thought or even explain what was going on because I didn't know what was happening. I was so medicated, I just started to sob and told him, "Don't do this, get out, and please don't come back." As if that scene with Zeus wasn't weird enough, and I mean Salvador Dali weird, read on! I had told the nurses earlier that there would be no more visitors. Yes, my soon-to-be ex-husband got in despite the signage, and thought I needed socialization at that point because I was just "depressed" and took it upon himself to remove the sign on his way out. I had it put back up; I didn't want anyone seeing me in this state, and I couldn't manage any more visits from anyone.

This is where an advocate would have been valuable. I was fully ambulatory and could utilize all my faculties on command July 31, 2007, and on August 1, 2007, just twenty-four hours later, I was laid out and couldn't move. I was so weak that I couldn't inch myself up with my feet, or feed myself. I could do nothing, period. The pain medicines weren't working properly, so they kept adding additional intravenous medications, which made it wild, to say the least. I should have been in the intensive care unit for a few days postoperatively to watch the flaps and myself, but I was on a medical surgical floor, which is not ideal for free-flap reconstruction. The point is, do not think for even a moment you can do this alone!

The physician ordered inpatient physical therapy for me at this point, to try to get me to move. I'll never forget it, I was so agitated, and this young physical therapist with a slight build came into my room with a walker. I lit him up verbally then threw him out of my room. I was awful, and I was sure the entire floor was drawing straws as to who was going to take care of me next.

The nurses could hear me swearing at this physical therapist, so they rush in, and were checking everything, saying to him, "Why don't you come back later?" He literally sprints out the door. One of the nurses on the medical surgical floor was Jennifer. She came in to tell me I had a phone call, and put the phone to my ear because I hadn't been able to pick up my cell phone, or charge it, for that matter. It was my ninety-year-old grandmother, Ginny, and my mother. My mom, God bless her soul, who knows there is no such thing as depression for me, said, "Cathy, listen to me. If you want to get out of the hospital, you have to make yourself move. I know you don't want too, or don't think you can. When I was in the hospital, I didn't want to do anything but lie there and die. My mother had an aneurysm in 1995 and has left side hemiplegia. Trust me, it's the only way out; you have to make yourself do it, will yourself to do it." She was right; that was exactly what I needed to do. Mother, thank you! I did need to move, I just didn't know how.

The nurse saw the bag, looked in, and commented on how darling the children were. She pulled everything out and put the pictures of the kids on the stand right in front of me and pinned up the crown my daughter had made me on the bulletin board. She read me Stephie's card. (Stephie, thank you for that gift of love. It made all the difference in my wanting to rise up and take action that very second.) I stared at everything and thought, if you want to get out of here, Cathy, it's between you and God right now, and you have to do something different.

When what you're doing isn't working and getting you to the finish line, it is time to put a little variation into an unbelievable human scene and rework it to your liking. I was in a manhole at that time with the worst condition known to man. For those of you who don't know what that is, it's called Baboon Ass! That is where you are so raw that only the flies want to be your friend. I had an insufferable case of it too. I had spiraled down to the bottom, humiliated, thinking I was going to die from crying, because I literally couldn't do anything. So I decided that no matter what, I was going to discontinue the intravenous medication and go to oral pain medication. I was still sobbing, telling Jennifer, we had to do something different; I couldn't stay like this. I had two children who needed me, and whom I needed, and I had to get out of there. She said, "I'll call the doctor and get a muscle relaxer added to the medication list, and we'll start."

I said, "Call a hospital chaplain and get anyone available to sit with me until I can shift over and am not hallucinating any-more. Also, make sure they have a coat of armor. I don't want to have to beg for clemency at the same time or anytime after their visit." I was so drugged up, she knew I was in agony and beyond heartbroken. I was in the most unspeakable pain you could imagine, lying there not being able to take care of myself or my children.

I requested someone who was Lutheran, then on second thought, changed my request to whoever was first available. I waited, and about an hour later, a priest, Father Flanagan, showed up. Okay, I'm not a Catholic, but I needed a body at this juncture. This was awful, but I told him I was so high and was going to change the pain medication management, because if I didn't do something different, I would be in a skilled nursing sit-uation soon. He said, "Okay, what would you like to talk about?"

I said, "I play the guitar for a Lutheran church in their con-temporary praise and worship service and really enjoy it. Have you ever been to one?"

He said, "No!"

I asked, "Have you ever seen a service like that?"

He responded succinctly, "No!"

I asked him, "How can you be here as a priest and not have seen that?"

In his very Irish accent, he said he had just come from Ire-land and was visiting, and in Ireland, you can get murdered for doing that, so he just avoided it. I was laughing so hard at this, saying, "That makes sense!"

So while I was holding on by my fingernails in that manhole, letting the drugs clear my system, I was mentally up on my elbows, then I had my trunk up with one leg out of the manhole. Soon, I had both legs out, and I was right side up and walking. I prepared myself to get dressed and get the hell out of there. I was laughing my ass off because I was not seeing or talking to Jedidiah on the wall anymore or he to me, so I was thinking, okay, it is better. I kept it up, and on day five, I turned the corner: My head was clearing, and I felt like moving my body.

Several of the nurses came over to help me sit up in bed, and I went right back down, but that evening, I went from the bed, and sat in a chair. On day six, I was up, walking holding a therapist—a different one, much taller, and no walker. I heard screaming down the hall, with a lot of four letter words. Suddenly the nurses all ran into my room, as I was sitting in my chair after my workout with the new cute therapist, and they said, "Ms. Doughty?"

I said, "It's down the hall!"

They couldn't believe the difference and said that my physicians vouched for me, reiterating that my previous citizenship during my stay was not normal. I apologized to all of them for my behavior and shenanigans while there, and they all hugged me and were wonderful about everything.

Now I was finally day seven post op, and my breasts had been removed. I had seven drains and I was leaving the hospital, going home looking like I had been in the jungle wrestling with a Bengal tiger. Blisters on my back, face, and forehead because of the tape allergy. I had perspired through everything I brought with me because of the narcotics, and I wanted to shower. I looked like Swamp Thing at this point and didn't know how to get myself showered and cleaned up or if it could even be done that day. I left the hospital and walked in to my residence, where Liseth met me at the door, and Stephanie, the nurse my mother paid for, who was covering me during the nights and weekends. I asked Stephanie if she could help me shampoo my hair. She said, "Yes, sure, I would be glad to!" I leaned over the bathtub with her help, and she shampooed my hair, got me medicated, and in bed. Then she continually checked on me and awakened me for pain medication and emptied the drains.

Cancer Cat Tip:

Plan on going to a place and get your hair washed, blown dry, and styled for two to four weeks postoperatively until you have the remaining drains removed and you can get your arms up to shower and shampoo your hair on your own. It's not a lot of money out of pocket, and you will feel like a million bucks. Showering is difficult at first, and you will need assistance with the drains and drying yourself for a while, so make sure you have your drain logs in the bathroom ready to be filled out.

Stephanie was so helpful and wonderful during the evenings

she stayed with me. She told me she had had cancer and went through bilateral mastectomies with reconstruction as well as uterine cancer and a hysterectomy a few years back and was doing extremely well. She looked stunning, too, and was delightful to talk with at night when I found it difficult to sleep. She even drove up to my house in her awesome, and hot new Mercedes, obviously totally successful after her surgery and treatment. She looked great and understood how I felt, and she was very accommodating. If she had been with me in the hospital, the unmanaged pain, the hallucinations for hours on end, and the extreme behavior would not have occurred. She would have had it remedied immediately.

The good news was I was at home now, but with drains; they're such a drag. You will need them though until you get the fluids down to a certain level, then the surgeon will pull them out. I tried the neck drain holder, then tried pinning them— what a nightmare. You can't get up to go anywhere without assistance, so as usual, Miss Doughty, who has the patience of a gnat, said, "Forget this!" and summoned Liseth.

I decided I was going to inspect the surgical sites, so I walked to the mirror, and while looking at myself, I started to become overwhelmed at the sites, and what I had just been through. Then out of nowhere, my son, Tommie, not Liseth, came upstairs with an emergency. I was still naked, looking at myself, and he said, "Mom, where's my skateboard and my tractor? I can't find them, and I need you to help me." It came as a flash that my loved ones could care less what I looked like. They just wanted me to be their mother and be there for them, so I told him where to find his toys, and pointed out of the upstairs window to exactly where each one was hiding, and he went barreling downstairs to find them. (Thank you, Tommie! Your question jolted me back into the present and centered me right there.)

Liseth followed upstairs shortly. I asked her to go out and find me some sweatshirts with pockets on the inside. She left and came back with three of them. Cool, I could put the lower drains in the pockets, but I needed something for the upper ones because I wanted to go and get a fill in my expanders. I had a lot of large bras in my drawer, but I didn't fit in them because I had lost about nineteen pounds during the big surgery, and my expanders weren't filled at this point. Liseth said, "Do you want one of mine? They are *muy caliente*."

Remember, I was high on oral pain medicines and not the happiest person to deal with, and I responded with something like, "Please, Liseth, for crying out loud. I trained in a bra bigger than this!"

She promptly responded, "Do you want it or not?"

I said, "Give it to me." I grabbed it out of her hands. She followed me into the bathroom dressing area, and she got me outfitted so I could go out to my appointment looking amazing. I love her, she is just the best.

I went to get a fill in my expanders, but only on one side because I had a problem with the other flap, so it was not going to be filled. I had to get a couple more drains out. My surgeon thought I was a genius, and I was thrilled because I was in a mini skirt with a darling designer sweatshirt and looked stunning. (Thank you, Liseth for dressing me up and sending me out looking wonderful!)

Liseth managed my drains and treated my wounds after the big surgery during the day after I no longer needed a night nurse. She was taken back when she first saw everything—horrified, really, with the number of wounds that needed to be cared for and what it all looked like. She kept it together, though, and did an excellent job. I couldn't have done any of it without her. She told me many months later that she just went home and cried and couldn't believe what had happened to me. She never understood the depth of any of it, so the change was alarming for her too. She needed the money though, so she continued to love, care, and put up with all of us. Praise, God!

She was coming over at 6:00 am, and the kids' dad would drop the children off at my house for breakfast, go back to his apartment, get ready, come back over, and take them to school. Liseth would pick them up after school, prepare dinner, get homework started, feed them, and get them bathed, and their dad would pick them up at my house after work and take them back over to his apartment to sleep. We followed this same routine for weeks.

I had planned on going back to work four weeks postoperatively, but I was not in any shape for that. I went back six weeks postoperatively, and it was still too soon. You need a minimum of six weeks or longer if you can do it. I was worried about my vacation days because chemo was coming and I wasn't sure what would happen. I needed to keep us all payrolled and going until I reached the treatment finish line.

Prior to returning to work, I had a pre-chemotherapy and radiation consultation with my oncologist and radiation oncologist, who went through every risk and benefit and thoroughly disclosed the percentages that each therapy would provide to minimize a future risk for recurrence. My ninety-year-old grandmother phoned me later that evening as I was reviewing all of the information and asked me, "Cathy, if the probability of the riskier therapies will get you into single digits for nonrecurrence, will you carefully consider chemo even if it is a small percentage? I know you have familiarized yourself with the risks and benefits on both sides, but my thoughts are that the benefit to you over the long run will outweigh any immediate or future health risk." I told her I would give each therapy very calculated and equal-weighted consideration—not necessarily by the reduction percentage to risk of each therapy, but what it would yield collectively to move me to single digits, percentage wise, for nonrecurrence.

I returned to work six weeks after the big surgery, and it was great to see all of my colleagues, who were delightful. I circled back for some collaborative conversations with Smokin Hot, Cash, Magic Man, and our boss, the Commander. Got together with the Evil Twins with whom I had worked with for over a decade and who are very dear to me. What is it with me and multiples? I certainly attract them, and I'm not a Gemini, either. One of the Evil Twins has triplets, too. Cash, Smokin Hot, Magic Man and both Evil Twins did so many accommodating and wonderful things when I was going through this, and I thank each and every one of you for your humor and recommendations as I was preparing my forms, documents and decision criteria matrices. You made it a lot better for me in an inordinately difficult time.

So I was back at work and circling back with the oncologist to discuss further questions regarding adjuvant chemotherapy and reviewing expectations. I met the chemo nurses, who checked my veins, and both reiterated that the veins won't hold up and that I would need a port. My oncologist ordered a port to be inserted into my left arm. I went across the street to the hospital, and an interventional radiologist and his team of nurses hooked up the greatest cocktail. The port was inserted, and I went back to work the next day. Four days later, I returned to the infusion center for my first of four rounds of chemotherapy.

Cancer Cat Advice:

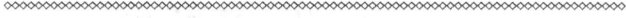

For most of us, it is extremely overwhelming to see ourselves for the first time postoperatively, even when we have carefully reviewed and calculated the impact of the surgical approaches previously. Do not become distressed. Remember, your wounds need time to heal, as do you, and that this is temporary. Everything will fade and look very different very soon. As the surgical sites close and the drains are removed, you will move on to the next phase. Also, carefully calculate the percentages that each therapy will offer you to move you closer to a reduced risk for recurrence.

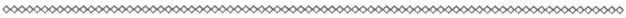

CHEMOTHERAPY AND
RADIATION TREATMENT

We'll start with chemotherapy first, since that is how I experienced it.

Now, I got dressed up for my first session of chemotherapy and every other one that followed. My cousin Cindy came over to my house dressed up too, and we drove together to the infusion center for my first round of chemotherapy. We were a couple of hot babes, dressed to the nines, walked in and couldn't believe what we saw: women sitting there without wigs or hair, quiet, some sad, in recliners and not talking. My cousin and I looked at each other and said, "So not us!"

We sat down and started going through all of our catalogs; we were shopping like crazy. Then the Pharm.D., came out to introduce herself to me and went through all of the drugs that were going to be infused into my body. She asked me my name, which checked—thank God and started to run the intravenous ondansetron (ZOFRAN®); then ran the docetaxel (Taxotere®), which took about two hours; followed by the cyclophosphamide (Cytoxan), which took about one and a half hours. I drank about four bottles of water while there and walked around. My cousin went to Starbucks and brought back a couple of espressos, and I was thinking, what is the big deal? Then we left.

I went to bed that night after infusion one still feeling good, but the next day, I woke up and I felt like the cockroach that just ate the Seven Dust. You know, the one on its back trying to scream, "Step on me!" The steroids were pulling on my fresh scars after surgery, and I felt horrible. Not nauseated—I was never nauseated. The aprepitant (EMEND®) worked beautifully, but I didn't feel like myself. Now, what do I do? I called my oncologists nurse, and she said this was normal. She advised me to take a half an Ativan and go to sleep and take the ibuprofen 800 mg as needed, so I did and went to bed. The next day, I was a little better, but not enough for my liking, and I was thinking I may not do anymore infusions.

However, as I started to wind down from the steroids, I was better, not so sped up, but I had to go to work, and it was my first working day post infusion. One thing I need to tell you, for me, each infusion was exactly the same: The effects were identical during the three weeks that lapsed in between. I never had what they call chemo brain. I was always on target, and I wrote everything down starting with the first infusion to cross-check and verify because I was working with numbers at the time.

Wigs, we haven't talked about them yet. Got to have them on your list once you hear that chemo is recommended. As a former chemo queen, believe me when I say this to you: With most of the chemotherapies, your hair is going to fall out. Not just the hair on your head, but on the rest of your body as well.

(Oddly, I still had to shave my legs though; I never could figure that one out!) Yes, it will fall out! Mine came out within twelve days of my first infusion. I was tugging on my hair thinking, "Oh, it won't come out. They're crazy." On day eleven, I could tug at my hair and nothing happened; on day twelve, I did the same thing and clumps came out in handfuls. When it happened, I was pacing back and forth for about ten seconds in my house. Then I reminded myself, "You control it; it doesn't control you!"

I called my stylist, went to the hair salon, walked into a private room, and got a cool flat top. I looked like my late father when he was alive, and my cousin Clif. Worked beautifully for what I needed, which was relief from hair falling out on me. My scalp didn't hurt anymore, and my wig fit beautifully. I had already gone to the wig shops earlier, tried on various wigs, and wrote down their brands, but I didn't buy any of them—the mark-up is unbelievable. Then I jumped on the Internet, Googled www.Joshua24.com, and ordered my wigs with a monofilament for twenty five percent of what the retailer wig shops were asking, and had them, shipped right to my house. I loved the Noriko brand, and my wig's names were Madison and Stacey. They were darling, and they held up great, too. My cousin Cindy would come over, and I would put them on, we'd get out the sangria, get a little lit, then she would go to work cutting and shaping them. They were so cute!

I would order a new one about every eight weeks. You will need to have a wig at your residence before you have your first infusion, so you are ready to put it on right after the first clump comes out and you cut it. If you don't want to go all the way down to the scalp, and I didn't when I had my hair cut down, tell your stylist. When my stylist turned on the clippers, my heart sank. I didn't cry though, but I did ask her to turn them off for a few seconds until I was ready. I asked her to use a number that would give me a flat top. Many people do a head shave, but I just wasn't ready for that. She turned me around away from the mirror and used the sheers that gave me the exact look I wanted. When she was finished, she turned me around, and I was absolutely fine, and I really liked it. If you prefer scarves with big earrings, caps, or nothing, that is absolutely up to you, but take care of yourself when your hair starts to come out so that it doesn't fall out on you. Generally, it is very unsettling for most people when this occurs.

I used my wigs all the time. I had to continue to look like I previously had professionally, so no one was the wiser. A little tip, Miss Doughty is passing onto you: Take advantage of www.Joshua24.com; they have really super deals. I had a wig burning ceremony when I took them off and quit wearing them. Approximately twenty weeks after the final chemo infusion, all of my hair came back beautifully.

Funny story with the little kids and wigs. One afternoon, I was home and got out of the shower, and the kids were in my room hiding. We used to play Where's My Chilis? They would hide somewhere upstairs, and I would count and come out yelling, "Where's my Chilis?" They were always giggling and moving around under the covers, so it was pretty easy to find them, but I would look around as if they were super hidden. I would gently pull the bed covers back and they would both be there curled up, and they would look at me, shocked! One time, Tommie said, "Mom, go get your hair back." Then simultaneously, Stephie said, "Mom, go get your wig." They had never seen me without my hair before. I told them that I would, but I reminded them, "It's still me, guys; don't be fooled by anyone's appearance."

I had a lot of surgery, the kids were over at their dad's at night, and I was working my ass off. Uncertain of anything but calm and hairless—both curtains and drapes, if you know what I mean. I was menopausal now too. The infusions had shut down my ovaries, so I was nonreproductive—that bothered me—more than losing my hair. And now my boss, the Commander, came into my office and declared that she didn't like the quality of one of the projects and didn't quite know what to do about it. You know one of those conversations you can't believe you're even hearing? I remained calm and said absolutely nothing except that there had been mitigating circumstances. I agreed to rework the project for her again. And I did, again and again and again until I finally decided I was out of there, by the end of the fiscal year. As it turned out, it would be before the end of the fiscal year.

I was very fatigued after chemotherapy and worked diligently because I had two kids and a mortgage, and radiation therapy was forthcoming. Except for the postoperative surgical time to recover, and the four vacation days I took off for the infusions because I was not sure if I was going to utilize, draw down or zero out my vacation bank, that was it. With radiation forthcoming, there was no guarantee whether I would be able to continue to work, so I just kept on going. However, if you weren't on the inside of my Posse, you would have never known what I was going through; I looked that good and kept myself together.

I need to elaborate here for a moment because one of the greatest professional experiences I had during this time was the opportunity to work with two extraordinary women who were doing very exciting, worthwhile work that made a difference daily in people's lives. Both women were physicians I knew and worked with in different capacities. One was my mentor and graduate advisor; the other I assisted, as her Black Belt, as she set up her ACE unit in the hospital. ACE, which stands for acute care for the elderly, specializes in geriatric care. One physician knew about my cancer; the other didn't. I absolutely loved every minute we worked together and the life-changing headway we made during that time frame. I remember talking with Dr. D. and asking her, "Where do the geriatrics go for exercise?" She exclaimed, "The pool!"

Dr. D., the one who didn't know about my cancer at the time, would be diagnosed with breast cancer herself two years later. I went to her immediately when I learned of it, because we now both worked for the same health science center. I told her the exact same things I am telling you. She is doing great, by the way, moving and shaking, making a difference in her faculty's and patients' lives with remarkable speed, and having a good time every single day of her life. I am so proud to know her!

Once the holidays were over and I had recovered from a staph infection I encountered after the port removal, I went to radiation planning to schedule my radiation treatment. Radiation therapy was a very straightforward process for me. I met with the radiation oncologist to discuss and determine the risks and benefits for my case. The radiation oncologist elaborated on all of my questions with very detailed and specific answers and had supporting publications to give to me for review. The radiation oncologist, along with the technologist, did a computed tomography study to determine where the lines would be, and I was marked with a permanent marker, which they sent home with me, so that I could touch up and highlight the lines as they faded. I was scheduled every morning at 7:00 a.m., so I could go right back to work following radiation.

I had thirty six treatments total, with boosts. I would come in with a French-pressed cup of coffee from the house, take my shirt off, and lie down, and they would start. My skin did burn, and I used aloe vera, which helped (there are other remedies you can discuss with your radiation oncologist as well, but that worked for me.) The skin turned red after approximately 15 treatments and blistered by the 29th session, but healed very quickly once radiation therapy was finished. I would apply two-by-two gauze pads, one with aloe vera and the other to hold it in place in my bra. Then when I showered, I would let the water fall upon my breasts, and the gauze pads would fall off and I would replace them with fresh ones following my shower. Radiation was easier for me than chemotherapy; I had more familiarity with it because of my professional experience in a Department of Diagnostic and Interventional Imaging. I was relieved when I started radiation therapy because I was nearing the treatment finish line.

Cancer Cat Tip:

This one's for those of you who have little kids who are spirited and always scheming like mine are. When they are misbehaving anywhere, but most especially in the car, you can tell them if they don't stop, you will take off your wig. All you have to do is to start lifting it up like you're going to take it off, and they will stop whatever they are doing that instant. They'll slide down to the floor of the car in their seatbelts, mind you, and hide!

THE ROOF CAVES IN

The day I finished radiation, I didn't even ring the bell, which is pretty customary for patients when they complete radiation therapy. I ran out of the place back to my car to drive to what I thought was mediation. I was finally ready to work out the details of and exit my failed marriage. You're not going to believe this; I went to this mediation meeting, and low and behold, it turned out that the attorneys had been retained by my soon-to-be ex-husband, who had filed for divorce thirty days prior. They had just held the waiver of notice, and I hadn't been formally served. Of course, Zeus neglected to mention the significance of that detail to me prior to the meeting, and as it was being announced in the meeting, said he didn't know, and then he stated that he did know. I was appalled at this unexpected revulsion, and immediately declared we were enemies. I may have declared a couple of other things, considering the circumstances. I left that ridiculous charade and retained an attorney.

Now I was dressed up, seriously dressed up with my hot wig, coat, jeans, and slides and walked as briskly as I ever had out of there. Then it dawned on me: Girlfriend, when you're flying by the seat of your pants (and I was, at that juncture), nothing sounds more official or reassuring than a Plan B. That's right; I needed to put Plan B., in place for this little event and for several others to follow. Once I left what I thought was media-tion, I immediately contacted one of my very dear friends who is an attorney for a renowned law firm here in Houston, TX. She gave me a referral to an outstanding attorney who handled the divorce with principled negotiation, always on the merits, and I was grateful.

Looking back, I was so disappointed at the time, not be-cause of the timing, the marriage had been doomed, and had been for some time with fault on both sides. But because I was weak and debilitated from all the therapies, my thoughts were that a little courtesy goes a long way.

Now, I was seriously concerned because the kids were with their father at night, and there were no orders in place or a Plan B finalized, for that matter. I had consulted with an attorney four months prior because the tension was insufferable, and the ad-vice was to finish the therapies. I was informed by legal counsel that the cancer could be used against me in a divorce proceeding if we were unable to settle. I waited, only to have what I thought was another unexpected bomb dropped on me. Little did I, or anyone else know, I would be living well, prosperous, victorious, having a joint visitation arrangement that I absolutely love, as do the children, with everyone thriving at the same time. The children have a good and loving father, and we do seven days on and seven days off, which works perfectly for everyone. All, hear me on this one: The best revenge is great living!

Sadly, almost half of marriages end in divorce. It is a common life transition that many people experience and thrive from; it can also occur for many people diagnosed with a degenerative disease, not just cancer. Don't think for a minute that you aren't beautiful and valuable—you are, even if others don't recognize it. You are not this body; this is not who, or what, you are. It is your essence or the life force that is your true identity. Don't doubt that for a second. What I have discovered during all of my cancer experience and all of the volunteer cancer coaching I have done since, is that it's fear. Plain and simple, indescribable, shrink-wrapped fear on their part. Hell, on your part, too. No one will give you a straight answer, so you are working through everything with a high level of uncertainty—which is reality—but it takes time to work through the misinformation you have been living with.

Bottom line: It is fear of caregiving and fear of financial ruin, period! No more, no less. You are still one hundred per-cent woman or man, and the essence of yourself is not attached to your body—please remember this, no matter what. At the time, I couldn't see the forest through the trees, another mis-representation. What I was unable to see, but did within a few days; for the children's father to have his freedom, mine would be forthcoming as well, so really it was the housekeeping before the party would get started.

I can verify this because I had doubts that were stalking me relentlessly until I talked to one of my very dear friends, Dr. Love, whom I have devoted an entire chapter too. I also wrote my own commercial that day after reading *Release Your Brilliance* by Simon T. Bailey, a great read and on my Recommended Reading List. I called it Cathy's Commercial, and I had it on my wall, in my wallet, and with me everywhere I went. It was to remind me that I was someone the world had never seen before and would never see the likes of again. I was a success as a mother, mentor, author, educator, clinician, and business leader and had a lot more work to do in service with others and in my lifetime. I reminded myself again and again that this experience was temporary, and as such, preparation and planning is a fundamental requirement throughout a cancer diagnosis, treatment and recovery. That I needed to continue without hesitation, regardless of what anyone's opinion of me was. At this point, I had been cut, drugged, burned, filed for divorce on, with reconstruction in-process, only to incur a first-class reduction in force, or "firing."

GETTING RIF'D OR FIRED REALLY AMOUNTS TO THE SAME THING: LACK OF REVENUE SOURCES

Remember my former boss, the Commander, from earlier in the story? Well, at this point in my recovery, I literally have three eyelashes and ten sprouts of hair left under my wig; my reconstruction was in process and not complete. My self-esteem had taken a major blow, and my boss phoned me and asked me to come over to the hospital straightaway. She said she needed to meet with me urgently. I had been working over at one of our rehab hospitals doing a project for the chief executive officer. I went to her office as requested, and when I entered the room, she handed me this letter. I opened it and read it to myself…with a quizzical smile on my face. It stated that, because of budgetary constraints, I and almost all of the rest of the Super Heroes had been selected for a reduction in force, or RIF. Isn't that a spiffy little term for getting fired? I read the letter, with a little smile intact, and when I was finished, I looked up at her with pursed lips and big eyes and just thought, "What a relief!" She asked, "Do you have any questions?"

I said, "No, um…I knew this could happen when I took the

job, and…so, no." I was out anyway at the end of the fiscal year. I knew that, but she didn't. She asked me, "What are you going to do?" I said, without appearing smug or overly exuberant, "Today, right now, I'm going home, and I am going to jump into a cold pool and celebrate!" And that's exactly what I did. I was so relieved.

Thankfully, at that point, I had finished my therapies but not the reconstruction work on my breasts, which for me was the most important part of the process. Now, having lost my job, I didn't have health insurance benefits unless I wanted to COBRA them, which I did. I had to; otherwise, the cost of the reconstruction would have been prohibitive and delayed. I had covered the family on my insurance; sometimes there was double coverage, but I had always over-insured to be certain the family was covered. Now that I had lost my job, I needed to pay almost $800.00 per month to keep myself and the kids covered and to keep an insurance policy intact that would finish the reconstruction phase, or else face an indefinite period of being "in process."

Cancer Cat Advice:

You have to stay up with all your health care benefits and where you are in your treatment phases and reconstruction, if it is in process. It takes long enough under normal circumstances, but if you don't manage your reconstruction, you can stay in a particular sort of incomplete state for an extended period of time. It would be to your advantage to think through the various stages of your treatment and recovery and make sure you have a plan that takes you all the way through..... and a back-up to the back-up plan. I hadn't envisioned or accounted for losing my job and my health insurance or being divorced before my treatment and reconstruction was complete, but it happened, and I needed a risk or contingency plan. It will be to your advantage to prepare your risk plan and insert a spending plan that includes all your revenue streams, expenses, and any reserves. Rework as often as necessary for each phase of your treatment should you experience a status change such as your employment, marital status, or any other associated funding sources. You will need to accumulate enough funds to account for the unexpected because there are a lot of unknowns when you are dealing with a cancer diagnosis and treatment planning. Additionally, know the location of all savings accounts, gold, or any other monetary reserves you can get access to should you need to liquidate them to cover interim expenses. Be prepared to stop all drafts out of your bank accounts until you can balance your expenses against your revenue streams. Remember, none of this is permanent; you can and will reverse all of this beyond your wildest imagination.

<u>CONTROL</u>

The first four phases, <u>D</u>efine, <u>M</u>easure, <u>A</u>nalyze, and <u>Im</u>prove, are enlightening and interesting to live through, to say the least. Now, getting your life back and your circumstances under <u>C</u>ontrol is more work, but you can do hard things because you have just finished or will finish all of your therapies!

First of all, everything up to this point is done from the immediate perspective: surgery, chemo, and radiation, with reconstruction initiated or about to be, but may still be "in-process." The worst part was behind me. I just needed to finish up the reconstruction and get back to work, but I needed to recover from the therapies I had just incurred. I began thinking about how I was going to rebuild myself, and get everything back in <u>C</u>ontrol. It was important for me to reduce the possibility of recurrence, within my treatment plan. Equally important was that there would be no more special cause variation such as what I had just experienced, another misrepresentation. Losing my job was a blessing in disguise, but the timing left me feeling out of control. I felt like the roof was caving in. I had to remind myself (many times) that when a door or two…or three…close on you, lots of other windows open up and propel you to a whole new dimension within the prism of uncertainty. It does not make it an act of the future: It makes it an act of the present, extending itself forward.

Stay with me—it really gets good here. Also, you might want to go get some tissues; you're going to feel joy!

CONTROL

How will the gains from your Improve or implementation plan be sustained?

What is the critical to future success and breast cancer recurrence prevention?

- » Hormone suppression
- » Follow-up visits
- » Exercise
- » Nutrition
- » Recovery

RECOVERY

I was midway through my recovery when I paused to take stock. I had been fired, my divorce was pending, reconstruction was still "in process." My recovery was going well, but my reconstruction wasn't finished, so I had to continue my benefits via COBRA. I didn't feel safe telling anyone I had lost my job because of the pending divorce, so I continued getting up every morning as though I was preparing for work. I would drive my car to the local Starbucks for my morning coffee, drive around until the cup was empty, and then I would park my car on the roof of the office building down the street from my residence and walk home. I did all this crazy stuff for weeks so my very-soon-to-be ex-husband couldn't use the circumstance against me in the divorce. The only one who knew everything the entire time was Liseth, my nanny...oh, and my cousin, Cindy. I tried to keep my situation going and look as normal as possible so no one suspected that anything was amiss.

However, I was going to be out of funds in six weeks with payouts and vacation. But I had a slush 401K fund when I worked at my previous hospital that I was 100% vested in and had forgotten about, so I converted everything over to IRAs and cashed them as I needed them. I was running out of money fast because I had significant expenses from all of the surgeries, medications, attorney retainer fees, children's tuition, multiple other expenses....I was looking at debt beyond my wildest dreams at that point—and indentured servitude for the rest of my life. It was all too much, and if I had allowed myself to be swallowed up by the enormity of the situation, a less-than-prolific outcome could have resulted. But not this Cat, kids! Instead, I wrestled back Control of my life, and decided to take action and rebuild myself.

I felt like I was ninety years old but never looked it ever, so I decided I would put all the time I was wasting driving around with my cappuccino's to good use. I started going back to my local YMCA and decided to jump into a cold pool and do water aerobics. I want to encourage each of you to try and exercise throughout your treatment if you can. It won't be easy because you'll feel tired following treatments, and exercise will be the last thing on your mind. However, consider that gentle stretching, yoga, swimming, or a walk around the block will make a huge difference to your general well-being and certainly your state of mind. Water aerobics is an especially good form of exercise because it is gentle on joints, and you can take it as hard or soft as your body will allow. It uses all your muscle groups and builds strength all over.

At my YMCA, I was the only pediatric in the pool—it was all geriatrics, who, by the way, were a heck of a lot faster than

I was. That first day, I got in the pool, I was so weak, but I was jacked up on French-pressed coffee, something I started in chemo that works beautifully when you are fatigued but have to keep going. The buoyancy weights kept popping up, and when I started to jog in the pool, I fell completely backward. I had no idea that because I had expanders full of saline in my chest I was really kind of hollow. It was difficult for me to find my balance, but I stuck with it. I focused on one gentleman (who looked about eighty-nine) and I decided my goal was to be faster than the slowest geriatric—he was my guy.

Initially he was substantially faster than me, but I was sticking with it because I had to gain some body strength. With the stress of my job gone, I could focus on rebuilding, not just my body but my life! I had to get to the bottom of C. Doughty. No easy undertaking for anyone, least of all me. I began scheduling appointments with nutritional specialists, estheticians, and a massage therapist, whom we'll call the Kahuna Ha-Ha.

THE KAHUNA HA-HA

My skin and body suffered as much as my hair, and while my hair didn't completely fall out, I had ten sprouts in the end. It certainly looked ashen and old. I started wearing concealer under my eyes and basically around my entire face during chemotherapy, and it worked well; I wear it to this day. My neighbor, is a producer for a network, and said all the news people use it. It is called gloCamouflage by gloMinerals, and it worked the best. It provided flawless concealment so no one ever guessed I had circles under my eyes from not sleeping. While I was at the spa picking up some more concealer, I asked about a massage and if they could schedule one right then. Lo and behold, this massage therapist walked out and said, "Hi, come with me!" I walked with her, talked to her and filled her in on what had happened. She listened attentively, intuitively understanding every word I was telling her, and without alarm.

I started laughing and told her I had just gotten out of a manhole with an acute case of Baboon Ass, which, by the way, is still in my opinion the worst condition known to mankind, and that I just wanted to feel better—like I did before all this cancer crap happened. She asked me to undress and slide onto her workbench. In a sudden fit of modesty, I told her I was leaving my underwear on, she said that was fine.

Then I told her I couldn't lie on my stomach because I had expanders in and they were like croquet balls: hard and uncomfortable. She said, "No problem. We'll do it on your sides; I will rotate you when I need to. Just relax."

She leaned me over and propped me up with pillows, and very gently, with great care, began to work on me. I started to feel my worries melt away and within minutes, I was relaxed and complete putty in her hands. She turned me over on the other side and continued to work her magic. I was just about to fall into a deep sleep because I was fatigued beyond belief, when she nudged me and said, "You ready?" Not really, I thought, but I got up, and she escorted me to this luxury shower where I stood and sat while I washed away all of the healing oils she had rubbed into my skin and muscles. She brought me some lemon water and reminded me to drink more clear fluids for the rest of the day. "Come and see me again in three days," she insisted.

"OK, I said!" What the heck, I was just about completely broke and featuring the Bangladesh Plan. I was just about out of funds, but I had to get myself back together, so I saw this as an investment and booked several other appointments for ninety minutes with her.

Along with my water aerobics, I continued to receive these therapeutic massages, and lo and behold, three weeks later, I was in the pool and found myself tied with the slowest geriatric jog-ging in the pool. I couldn't believe what a difference just a few weeks had made. Here was the actual test though. That Thursday was the end-of-school pool party for my children, and I had committed to going. I found a dive skin, which is an aquatic suit that made me look like Wonder Woman…well, it was red and blue, and that's about where the similarities end. This aquatic suit covered me from neck to ankle, and down to each wrist. It was really cool because I had been radiated and I was not up for any sun on my already burned and blistered skin. When it came time for the party, I just wanted to dive into the pool and play with my kids. I didn't want to have to explain anything to anybody…the less people saw, the better. While there, the kids talked me into going on the waterslide with them. Initially, I was panicked because I was really afraid of getting hurt, but at the same time, I wanted to see if I could do it. I climbed up the stairs using all my lower body strength and got up there right behind my son. It was when I was up on the tube slide ladder, with my legs in the tube, that I freaked out because I was thinking, "Holy Smokes, Cathy! What are you doing? You're going to be stuck like Shamu, and they're going to have to call the local fire department to get you out with a cherry picker or crane."

Then I remembered how strong I had felt in the pool the day before, and I grabbed onto the sides of the tube chute and amazingly pushed my body off into the pool, laughing out loud underwater and giving one thousand different types of thanks for this new strength. I owed it all to Bert! You see, Bert, which is short for Berta, is what I call a Kahuna Ha-Ha.

Berta is an expert in diagnosing illnesses and then applying her craft as a masseuse to rehabilitate the body. She is particularly good at massaging the affected body parts with specific therapies that rejuvenate and assist the body in recovering from cancer treatments, which are grueling but all we have at this juncture in time.

Cancer Cat Advice:

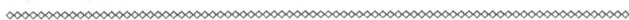

If you are in Houston, you can look her up at www.MassagebyBerta.com, or if you are visiting Houston and need a Kahuna Ha-Ha with superior touch capabilities, make an appointment! You can do it through her website, and it's the living end. I continue to see her to this very day and highly recommend her or one just like her. If you can't schedule time with Berta, find a masseuse in your area who can offer the same complement of healing remedies.

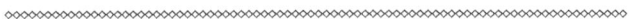

DR. LOVE'S PSYCHO SALVATION

I have mentioned Dr. Love earlier throughout this book. We have never been involved, but have a friendship which consists of mutual love and respect that transcends just about everything. I have known Dr. Love for years, played guitar with him weekly, talked with him frequently, and then sometimes not at all for long stretches at a time, but the bond is always there.

As a matter of fact, when I was originally diagnosed, he called and told me about what had happened with his sister Patti. She had also been diagnosed with breast cancer, and had a mastectomy. He put the two of us in touch with one another, and it was a very soothing conversation and moment for me when she shared her experience with me. She thoughtfully checked in on me during my surgeries, treatments, and recovery. It was all very reassuring, because when you're falling deeper and deeper into the prism of uncertainty, and the misrepresentation of the information becomes overwhelming, you need to talk with others who have been through it, and came out on the other side whole and strong. Patti was all that, and it centered me every time we talked.

Honestly, I found that the more I visited with those who

had made it to the other side, the more energy, motivation, and enthusiasm I accumulated. This is just as important as anything else you may do for yourself, and when you get to the other side, be sure to talk with anyone needing your experience. I made it to the other side, and by all accounts, I am thriving and am 100% available to gab about anything and everything regarding breast cancer.

There is a lot to Dr. Love, but I'll be brief (a saying I shop-lifted from him). I had my port removed after chemo during December 2007, six days before Christmas. Unbeknownst to me, a microbe had broken off during the removal and landed on one of the expanders, and I had a staph infection. Three days later, I couldn't move, and I mean, could not move. I had a fever, and the entire right breast was inflamed, red, and swollen. I was shaking uncontrollably and called the kid's dad to tell him I was going to have to send the kids over to him because I was under the weather. It occurred to me that I had an infection, and I got myself to the plastic surgeon, who confirmed that indeed it was an infection and I would be admitted to the hospital for at least five days. He also said I may lose the expanders if the antibiotic infusion didn't clear it up. I could not believe what I was hearing or what was happening to me, and was too sick to ponder that possibility.

I was also too sick to be scared, and I tried to convince myself it would all work out. I found myself at the hospital in a treatment room six days before Christmas. The hospital staff was kind enough to give me VIP status and started the antibiotic infusion promptly. I was lying in the hospital bed, all connected with a new I.V., after just having the port removed permanently, and was feeling very low when my mobile phone rang. It was Dr. Love.

I didn't tell him what was happening at the time because it was so wonderful to hear his voice. We just talked and laughed about anything and everything. We have such a similar sense of humor. On one level, we're somewhere between the ages of eight and eleven, so you can imagine what cracks us up—just about everything. That call was a lifesaver, and I was so grateful to have him on the other end. It would be months later before I told him how much that call meant to me and what was going on at the time. I will share that my feelings for him are visceral and transcended anything earthly I have ever known in my friend-ships with other men. I have the highest regard and respect for his presence in my life.

It was six days before Christmas in 2007, and there I was in a damn hospital bed. My son's birthday is December 28th, and as I do every year, I had everything ready to pull down from the attic with ease. "Thank God, I am so organized," was all I could think about as I lie there being infused with daptomycin for five days and singing Christmas carols to myself until I was really fed up.

When I was finally released, I drove myself home, got down on all fours and kissed the carpet on the stairs of my residence and began cooking Christmas dinner for my cousin, her family, and my kids. Nobody knew what I had just been through, and when my cousin found out, she nearly strangled me. Christmas Eve dinner was great, by the way, and we had a wonderful time. Later that night, I went over to my neighbor's house after the kids fell asleep, and I asked their son, Grant, if he would help me pull out the presents and bring them down from the attic for the kids to open Christmas morning, and he did.

Upon reflection, that whole infusion thing might not have gone so well had Dr. Love's Psycho Salvation not come across the wire at that exact moment, enabling me to call up my energy and focus on my healing so I could get the heck out of there without having to endure further surgery.

Cancer Cat Advice:

Surround yourself with people who lift you up and inspire you to laugh, love, and live! Dr. Love and I continue to visit frequently and keep up with one another's shenanigans and discuss how each of us needs a handler because we're having such a good time. He was there for me—unknowingly at times—and it made a huge difference.

HAVING A GOOD TIME LIVING
LIFE THROUGH THE PRISM
OF UNCERTAINTY

Here is how it all turned out! Yes, I was RIF'd, but within a week of being released, I had three job offers, three really incredible job offers. I picked the one I thought would yield the greatest job satisfaction. In the end, I joined an academic medical school, and finished my own physical rehabilitation. I changed plastic surgeons because I wanted experimental implants for the final exchange in my reconstruction process. I scheduled the INAMED 410 experimental implants exchange surgery two weeks before I was to begin my new job on July 7th, 2008.

Following the implant exchange surgery, I contracted the plastic surgeon's nurse to stay with me postoperatively and had not one issue at any time. I now have smoking-hot, gorgeous full C-cup breasts that will stop a train! They are absolutely beautiful. I look great and am very comfortable with the permanent implants. By the time I started my new position, I had been divorced three days, my implants were just two weeks old, my hair was a little short, and I was sure some people were thinking, "Hmmm...What's up with this new person?" I had interviewed for the position in a gorgeous Noriko monofilament wig named Madison that was so convincing, you couldn't tell it wasn't my real hair.

From that first day on the job, I have loved my work and have been proud of my decision to join the institution. I finished my master's degree in May 2008, right before I went back to work. I remember meeting one of the nurses who was getting my I.V. ready when I had the final exchange for the permanent implants. When I told her what I was doing, she revealed to me that she was a breast cancer survivor and finished her Master of Science in Nursing during her treatment. I was pleased to hear this as I had received so much resistance from people telling me "School, spool!" to which I replied, "Without increased expertise, you can't get increased financing!" I have always been a proponent of higher education and will be all the days of my life. To me, it makes such a difference, and to be honest, having something completely separate from my cancer treatment kept me sane.

When the kids' dad and I finally severed our marriage on July 3, 2008, we decided on a seven-day-on/seven-day-off schedule with the children. This arrangement makes it easy for our children to go back and forth to each parent's home without difficulty because we live virtually five miles from one another. Because we did not do a traditional arrangement, there is no subsidy for either parent. At the time of being RIF'd and the divorce being finalized, as head of household, I definitely needed to generate additional revenue streams or change my standard of living.

Know this, my friends: Poverty and Miss Doughty are not compatible—never have been and never will be. Even after I returned to work full-time, I felt I needed to generate additional income to rebuild my pension and savings, which had been depleted during my treatment. I had met with my academic advisor for informational advice and counsel prior to returning to work. She was extremely helpful and sent me to meet one of her colleagues, who told me about the fascinating world of asynchronous learning environments. I did some research and began applying as an associate faculty member for other universities in the online teaching arena. I do this on a part-time basis, which I find very rewarding, and it works beautifully, because I work full-time and need to be on campus. I didn't want another job where I would have to leave the children. Virtual classrooms go on 24/7/365, so when I am finished with my full-time responsibilities and the children are in bed, I work with my collegiate student body.

I successfully refinanced the house and pulled out just enough cash to cover the family until I could recreate the new revenue streams and continue to keep all of us in the property where I brought the kids home from the hospital. That was my rationale for taking on part-time work in the beginning. I could have started over somewhere else, but the thought of moving at that time, with all that had occurred and was about to occur, was just physically and emotionally overwhelming. Moreover, I didn't want the kids to have a traditional visitation arrangement, nor did their father. We both wanted to be present in the children's lives, so this was a mutual agreement, and it has worked very well for everyone.

RECONSTRUCTION COMPLETE

I had both nipples constructed during a lunch break within months of receiving my new implants, and was very happy with the cosmesis. Going to get them colored or tattooed was a completely different experience. Stay tuned; this is funny!

Nipples were healed and ready to have the permanent make up or tattooing applied for coloring. I had gone to another plastic surgeon's office, because the service was not available with my other plastic surgeon. I walked in and was greeted, taken back into a large room, and introduced to a medical assistant, who talked with me about what I would like. I explained exactly how I would like them to look, and she asked me if I would like a shot of morphine. I explained that I would not; I don't tolerate morphine well, and that it makes me vomit. "Would you like some wine?" she asked.

"Absolutely, that I would love!" I said.

She came out with a bottle of chardonnay and poured me a full glass of wine in crystal stemware. I removed my blouse, and she went to work. She told me she really needed some music to get into this; classical music was playing, but she needed some rock. I said, "Classic rock is my favorite."

She asked, "How about the Rolling Stones?"

"Fabulous!" I exclaimed.

She put it on, then it went to Led Zeppelin, and three hours later, viola, I was drunk and done! Looking good, feeling great! My ride raised her eyebrow because I am not much of a drinker, but for this, I was. She took me home, gave me two ibuprofen, and I walked upstairs with a Cheshire Cat grin—so happy. I jumped into my bed and went to sleep, cracking up because I was completely finished and felt so darn good!

FINDING INSPIRATION IN
MUSIC AND KIDS

The fall and winter of 2008 were wonderful. I had successfully taken back control of my situation and was gainfully employed again. I continued to play guitar throughout it all, which
was a huge source of pleasure for me. Playing at Sunday praise
and worship services and attending Sunday school are both very
important social activities for me and very healing. As I mentioned earlier, I am a kid at heart, so being able to play music for
friends and families in the course of worship is a lot of fun and
extremely rewarding. During Christmas of 2008, our Sunday
school class went out caroling in the neighborhood and at the
Faith House, and I was deliriously happy to be able to partici-
pate.

The Faith House is an outreach program that offers patients
and their families a place to stay while they are going through
cancer treatments, transplantations, etc. The Faith Alive band,
and other members from the congregation were all out that
night. I was playing acoustic guitar, and we just started walking in the neighborhood and around the Faith House, playing
and singing, big time. Everyone who saw us—all of our children

were out in front, singing their hearts out—asked us to come into their homes, where they gave us cookies, drinks, anything and everything.

When we finished, we went back over to the Faith House, and the little kids were in front of me again. We knocked on one of the apartment doors, and a man opened the door and stood there with his young son, who was quite clearly going through some very debilitating therapies. His son was very weak and shaking, but curious. He held out his hand, and all of the children reached for it, they grabbed the boys' hand and arm, and he theirs, then he stopped shaking and just smiled with jubilation. I will never forget the magic that happened during that night, and I thought back to what it was like the year before, when I was singing Christmas carols to myself in a hospital room. What a marvelous experience it was to be in the presence of this boy and his father with everyone, smiling and holding hands, surrounded with love. Thank you, kids for what you all did that evening for that youngster, his family, yourselves, and everyone else you touched that night. Your influence was further than your reach.

Everyday, I give thanks for everything that crosses my path. I am deliriously and magnificently happy, having a good time, feeling great, and looking hot. I don't know what's on the other side of this life, but whatever it is, I hope it is as good as what I have experienced so far and the lessons I have learned as the prism refracts another dimension in my life to learn from.

As a result of my cancer experience, I became a better mother, educator, author, business leader, clinician, mentor, cousin, and friend. I have utilized all of the lessons in my cancer coaching with others and speaking with newly diagnosed patients and their families who are experiencing cancer and trauma. I always remind them: You survived and have been spared. The body did its job and recovered itself. Don't relive things from the past; just know that if it weren't for those problems, you would never have risen above the level you were at. Remember the angel sitting next to me when I was fit for a straightjacket—encouraging me to stay in the moment?

You survived the treatment plan, and now it's time for you to figure out your purpose. I know mine, and I continue to live it every day. For me, a good time is when I am loving, not being loved or seeking love, but just loving either my loved ones, friends, work, or others. It is also watching you having a good time everyday you live your life through the prism of uncertainty. I used to be so fearful of looking at uncertainty, when it dawned on me that it has been this way from the beginning, and it's a much sexier way to live because right now is all you've got, so you need to have a rocking hot good time. I want to leave you with this: If any piece of my story has helped you and made your journey with cancer any easier, it was all worth it.

Remember, I love all of you, and we need to keep the pressure on medical research and science to work hard and fast to design this disease out of existence. Please drop me a line and let me know how you are doing or impart any advice and tips you have discovered. I always want to hear what you are up to, and how you're having a good time!

I love you all. Thank you, and God Bless!

–*Cathy*

EPILOGUE

I wanted to let you know how everybody is doing.

Cindy is married to a drop-dead gorgeous and successful oil and gas man. They live all over the world, so she's having a good time!

Dr. Love continues to play guitar and teach students in Houston, TX. He is thriving; and always scheming up something wild and crazy, so he's having a good time!

Ginny, my ninety-three-year-old grandmother, who still plays bridge weekly, drives and does whatever she pleases is having a good time!

Liseth sent her son Joey to the first grade this year, and he will be in the Gifted and Talented program at his elementary school. She says she's still having a good time working for me, go figure. I just love her!

Molly is selling real estate, making bank every day, and loving her seven grandchildren. The relationship is so natural because they all have a common enemy, their parents, which are her children, so she's having a good time!

Steve and Nikki are living out in Southern California, raising my niece and nephews, and it is always some kind of hilarious shennibooboos with those guys. Nikki is healthy and well, and they are both earning and burning, and crazy about their family and are having a good time!

Tom and Libby are living out in Southern California, working and tending to my other twin niece and nephew. They're both working hard snapping necks and cashing checks, crazy about their family too, and having a good time!

The Kahuna Ha-Ha, Berta, is working and continues to provide healing and recovering therapies to those seeking well-being here in Houston, and is having a good time!

Zeus remarried and bought a house in Bellaire, Texas, and looks like he's having a good time!

THE SUPER HEROES

Cash just gave birth to her twin sons, Jack and Jett, and is busy with double bottles, double strollers, double diapers, and double, double, double everything. She waited forever for these boys and found a whole new way to love and is having a good time.

Smokin' Hot got married, got promoted, and is working as a director at a large hospital in Houston, having a good time.

Magic Man moved and went to work for the Mayo Clinic. He and his gorgeous wife have two beautiful daughters, so he is surrounded with women—totally having a good time!

The Evil Twins, both of them named Rich, work for me. They're both having the time of their lives with their families. They remind me daily that they have to keep the books for a full year when their working with me to make sure they're having a good time! You two, honestly!

ABOUT THE AUTHOR

Catherine Doughty, MS, CCHI, holds a Master of Science in Bioinformatics from The University of Texas School of Biomedical Informatics. In addition to her career as Director for the Department of Diagnostic and Interventional Imaging, she is a trained Lean Six Sigma Black Belt. She also serves as an Adjunct Associate Professor for three universities. For the first time in book form, Cathy provides an intensive understanding and step-by-step guide utilizing scientific methodology to navigate complex issues and medical decision making in an uncertain decision space that a patient experiences during a cancer diagnosis and treatment planning. Her personal experience, paired with her sense of humor, is woven throughout this book and provides insights on how to utilize a tool set and see how information being refracted can be misrepresented through the prism of uncertainty. She will walk you through everything with decision matrices, forms, and discussion documents while keeping you intact, on the edge of your seat, and empowered through every page.

RECOMMENDED READING

Kris Carr; *Crazy Sexy Cancer Tips*, 2007; www.Crazysexycancer.com

Simon Bailey; *Release Your Brilliance*, 2008; Harpers & Collins

Larry Burkett; *Nothing to Fear*, 2003; Moody Publishers, Chicago

Fran Drescher; *Cancer Schmancer*, 2002; Warner Books

Peter S. Pande, Robert P. Neuman, Roland R. Cavanagh; *The Six Sigma Way – Team Fieldbook*; An Implementation Guide for Process Improvement Teams; 2002; McGraw-Hill

Ann E. Frahm; *The Cancer Battle Plan*; 1997, Penguin Putnam

INDEX

www.ingramcontent.com/pod-product-compliance
Lightning Source LLC
Chambersburg PA
CBHW060906280326
41934CB00007B/1205